In Praise of]

When a 21st century woman is preparing... lot of research. She takes a course, reads textbooks and sees many medical practitioners. But dwarfing all of these in importance, the most critical source of birth wisdom is other women's birth stories. Nothing else comes even close in terms of value, relevance and meaningfulness. But then there's a problem: For one reason or another, the women who had traumatic, unusual, or complicated births seem to get all the limelight. Those are the stories that appear in the media, that get focused on in the textbooks, that are repeated in hushed whispers during coffee mornings. What we could do with hearing are the great yet normal ones, the ones that went as nature intended, the ones that women have been capable of and pulling off since the dawn of the species. So that's why the book is needed. Why is Caroline the woman to write it? That's simple inspiration.

Lots of people do amazing things. Only a few of them can also inspire those around them to do amazing things as well Caroline is one of those. Caroline's voice is inspirational, without any condescension or gimmickry. She has told her own birth experiences in a way that feels relevant to any expectant mother, and she has collected other voices and stories that complement hers. In an age when we no longer grow up in a tribe that preserves and continuously passes on a collective maternal wisdom, this book is a must.

Dina Westenholz-Smith,
Mum of three, Magistrate

We are still relying on 1970s American texts to bring words of inspiration for pregnant and birthing women. I see a lot of mums to be in my practice as a herbalist and am so pleased at the thought of having your book as a tool to inspire them along their journey. I held the stories I'd read and from those women around me to help me through my pregnancy free of fear at the thought of birth....I'm sure this lead me to a positive outcome at the end of it....thank you so much for writing this valuable tool.

Fiona Heckels, Herbalist, Dorset

Caroline Murray is a passionate advocate of birth as it should be. I commend her dedication to supporting and empowering women through her work.

Lucy Pearce, contributing editor JUNO magazine, Birthing from Within mentor and mother of three

This book will fill a definite gap in the Market and make an essential contribution to promoting natural birth as a real possibility for all women. I will definitely buy this book and looked high and low for something similar as the birth of my second child approached last year.

Mother of 2, south London

I have had the pleasure and the privilege of being the author's midwife since the beginning of her first pregnancy and I believe she is the most qualified person to have written this book, it will become a "must have" on the reading list of every woman who has ever thought about having a baby naturally, a straightforward natural approach to a straightforward natural event. I will recommend it to every woman planning a natural birth that I come into contact with.

Katrina Caslake, Yours Maternally Independent Midwifery, mother of 2 and grandmother

Thank you Caroline for taking the time to create your book it is so needed in today's hurried time conscious, society, space to think about the beauty and miracle that having babies is. During both my pregnancies I was inspired by reading other women's stories of natural, gentle birth.

These stories kept strength in my heart during the darkest moments of my labours.

Karen White, Herbalist, Mother of 2

Caroline Murray has written the book that is missing from the mainstream market. A book that contains real, success stories from women who have chosen home births and have enjoyed and benefited from that experience. While there are books 'out there', which present home birth from a professional's point of view, as one of the options available to women today, there is a distinct lack of real stories of unproblematic, gentle, easeful and even ecstatic, in their essence, home births, written from the point of view of the woman. These are the kind of stories very much needed in our culture today and the ones other women need to hear and be inspired by. This gap is bridged by this book.

Dafni Milioni, Ph.D, Counselling Psychologist and Yoga teacher, mother to two homebirthed children

Natural Birth in a Nutshell

Caroline Murray
with Midwife, Katrina Caslake

AUTHORS PLACE
—PRESS—

Published by Authors Place Press
9885 Wyecliff Drive, Suite 200
Highlands Ranch, CO 80126
AuthorsPlace.com

Copyright 2019 © by Caroline Murray

All Rights Reserved

No part of this book may be reproduced or transmitted in any form by any means: graphic, electronic, or mechanical, including photocopying, recording, taping or by any information storage or retrieval system without permission, in writing, from the authors, except for the inclusion of brief quotations in a review, article, book, or academic paper. The authors and publisher of this book and the associated materials have used their best efforts in preparing this material. The authors and publisher make no representations or warranties with respect to accuracy, applicability, fitness or completeness of the contents of this material. They disclaim any warranties expressed or implied, merchantability, or fitness for any particular purpose. The authors and publisher shall in no event be held liable for any loss or other damages, including but not limited to special, incidental, consequential, or other damages. If you have any questions or concerns, the advice of a competent professional should be sought.

Manufactured in the United States of America.

ISBN: 978-1-62865-606-0

Contents

ACKNOWLEDGEMENTS **11**
PREFACE **12**
INTRODUCTION **15**

PART ONE 17

CHAPTER ONE **18**
SO, YOU'RE PREGNANT

CHAPTER TWO **25**
NATURAL vs. MEDICAL

CHAPTER THREE **30**
PREPARE YOURSELF

CHAPTER FOUR **38**
LOOKING AFTER NO. 1

CHAPTER FIVE **43**
PMA: POSITIVE MENTAL ATTITUDE

CHAPTER SIX **45**
LOOKING AFTER NO. 2 (THE MAN IN YOUR LIFE)

CHAPTER SEVEN **48**
THIS IS IT! LABOUR AND BIRTH

CHAPTER EIGHT... **62**
JUST IN CASE – MEDICAL INFORMATION AND TERMINOLOGY

CHAPTER NINE.. **65**
ONWARD INTO MOTHERHOOD

PART TWO 70
APPENDIX... **94**
RESOURCES **96**
ABOUT THE AUTHOR **99**

To Mum and Dad,
for giving me the gift of life

For Naomi, Hannah, Leila & Joseph

"Just as a woman's heart knows how and when to pump, her lungs to inhale, and her hand to pull back from fire, so she knows when and how to give birth."

Virginia Di Orio

ACKNOWLEDGEMENTS

I would like to thank Guru Ram Kaur, my Kundalini Yoga Teacher for whom I began to write this as a workshop. Anne Tison for pregnancy yoga, Guru Kaur for notes and all round inspiration, Melanie Goose for superb and ruthless editing, Saffia Farr and Lucy Pearce at Juno Magazine for their ongoing support with my writing and various projects, my husband for everything. Without him, truly none of this could have happened.

"Like a friend telling you how it is, this book is very straightforward and speaks a wealth of truth about pregnancy and birth, gleaned from the author's own experience."

"Made me feel like getting pregnant all over again, simply to experience it from this lovely and positive perspective."

"I wish I had read this book when I had my first baby. It could have saved a lot of grief."

"The author actually cares about expectant mothers as women in their own right going through a life-changing experience."

"Easy to read, down to earth, sound, practical advice for first, second, third (or more) time mothers."

"Makes natural birth seem like the most normal and, well, natural, thing in the world."

"The book every thinking mother-to-be is reading."

PREFACE

My mother bore me, although in hospital, naturally, and with little fuss. She stayed at home to bring us up, cooked good wholesome food, and encouraged us to think independently and to enjoy the outdoors. My father is an inspired doctor who doesn't believe in drugs (although occasionally prescribes champagne). My grandfather on my mother's side (Grandpa Sid) was amongst the first to adopt vegetarianism in England, and practiced yoga. He died when I was eighteen years old and I inherited a number of yoga books and some years later found a class and began to practice. I continued to be interested in health, good food and yoga. With hindsight, it's very easy to see how my life had prepared me to go on and have natural births. I had been raised with a number of the necessaries. But don't worry if you're upbringing sounds miles away from this: that's why I've written this book! And anyway, I still had more to learn.

Until I was about thirty years old, I lived my life on whims, went with the flow, and didn't really think much about it. So, when, at the age of 30 I found myself in a depression, and not at all where I wanted to be, began to think very deeply about my life, my goals and aspirations, and particularly whether or not I wanted to have children. Up until that point, I hadn't really been sure about any of it. I started to read self-help books, usually chosen from a bookshop shelf when I was in need of inspiration. Books such as The Purpose of Your Life by Carol Adrienne and The Artist's Way by Julia Cameron came my way. They started to make me realise that I was the master (or mistress) of my own destiny.

It was then that I decided I really did want children, and I had better find a decent man to have them with. This wasn't a question of sperm donation. I needed someone who I could be in partnership with, to share this journey of parenthood, and of life.

So, I focused on developing my own life, becoming more myself, and learning to be vibrant again. Along the way I opened myself to the possibility of meeting this man. Yoga was a constant thread, giving me the tools to learn to breathe, be still and listen to my inner voice. I was brought to a state where I was consciously living my life. I was the driver, not the passenger, and this is where I found myself when I became pregnant with my first baby. I did not want to be a passenger of the medical services, delivering my baby to me, in their way. I wanted to be the driver of my birth experience, choosing how, where and with whom I would birth my baby.

I had learnt that by developing clarity on something I deeply desired, I could attract it to me by focusing on it in an intensely positive way. These were the skills and thought processes I employed when planning my births. Sometimes, obstacles would arise, usually borne out of previous experiences, assumptions, fears, or outside sources. Keeping focused on a natural, beautiful birth is work in itself when we are surrounded by others telling us how awful it is, and images on TV which show only pain and suffering. But, this was the key to my natural births: to zone out from the external stuff, and tune in to my own instincts. Sometimes stuff would come up from within myself, fears about whether or not I could do it, the pain; did I actually believe I was having a baby. I found that if I looked at these fears, voiced them to my husband or my midwife, maybe wrote about them, the very act of shining a light on them would cause them to disappear or diminish. I could then continue to focus on the positive outcome I had envisaged: birthing my baby into the world naturally, peacefully and lovingly.

Much of the information I give you is inspired by my own wonderful midwife, who gave me the confidence and support to carry through my own wishes for my births. Having another woman just totally believe in you is incredibly powerful. I also attended pregnancy yoga classes to train my body and mind to open to the experience. Having a whole group of women behind you is also wonderful! Aside from that, I was encouraged by Ina-May Gaskin's Spiritual Midwifery,

Here, I'd like to share with you some of the things I've learned on my journey which I hope will help with yours. Birth is a miracle of life, a gift to be honoured and bathed in beauty. Come with me to make your birth one of the most beautiful experiences of your life.

INTRODUCTION

When I was pregnant with my first baby, it never occurred to me that my waters would break in an Indian restaurant but that's exactly what happened. I then proceeded to have a wonderful, peaceful labour and birth at home, followed over the next few years, by three further natural deliveries. But, what is this thing about natural childbirth? Are we women gluttons for punishment? You'd never catch a man saying, "I'd love to have a natural vasectomy" would you? So, why opt for a natural birth when there are effective and safe methods of pain relief? Even a caesarian these days is deemed as safe as giving birth vaginally. Perhaps I need to rephrase the question? Why opt for a medical birth when you can have a remarkable, empowering and brilliant experience?

Some years back, I did a parachute jump. For several weeks after the experience, I felt magnificent. I felt I could do anything, be anything. I was on top of the world. This is how I felt after birthing my babies and this is how I want you to feel too.

So, what do I classify as natural childbirth? Simple: a vaginal delivery with minimum intervention. Despite what you have probably heard, I am here to tell you that childbirth can be gentle, ecstatic, orgasmic and enjoyable. It is an enormous, life-changing, awe-inspiring happening that deserves attention, care and loving handling.

This book promises to:
1. To inform you about natural childbirth and your options
2. To empower you to take control of your birth experience

3. To inspire you towards a natural and wonderful birth and entry into motherhood

We have become as children on the issue of childbirth, by having all our knowledge taken away from us in the medicalisation process. Knowledge equals power. I hope that by sharing the knowledge that I have gained from my experiences, I can empower you to enjoy yours.

PART ONE

Chapter One

SO, YOU'RE PREGNANT

"A grand adventure is about to begin."
Winnie the Pooh

I REMEMBER BEING AT A PARTY when I was pregnant with my first daughter and women I had never met before came over to me, striking up conversations about motherhood, asking me about my pregnancy, and sharing their experiences. I couldn't remember another time in my life where I had felt so welcomed. Regardless of culture or nationality, the common link of motherhood connects you with other mothers wherever you are in the world. It's like a secret society that you didn't know existed until you joined. So, welcome to the club!

When you did the pregnancy test and saw the positive result, you probably experienced all sorts of mixed feelings alongside the joy and excitement. This is the beginning of a completely new phase for you and your partner, who will soon be becoming a family. You may be starting to feel differently about every aspect of your life: your body, your work, your relationship with your partner, your relationships with your family and friends. You may be thinking about when you'll going back to work, how you're going to care for your baby, maybe who's going to care for your baby. Often, during pregnancy people either move house or undertake household renovations as they begin to think about the kind of home they want to bring their baby into, and focus on 'nesting'. Maybe your pregnancy is the result of years of trying, or you may have conceived quickly. Whichever way, it is likely to be rocking your world in more ways than one. During my pregnancies I felt an incredible sense of peace with myself in the knowledge that I was doing something vital, and important.

Your body will be changing too, subtly at the beginning by gaining a few pounds in weight and having more tender breasts. You may notice your sense of smell and taste change, and that you start to dislike flavours which you had previously loved. I developed a dislike for pepper during my first pregnancy: it just tasted so strong and pungent in a way I had never noticed before. With the extra blood pumping around your body, you may feel warmer than usual I experienced my first winter of not ever feeling cold which was blissful.

As your pregnancy progresses until your belly is large and round (and beautiful), your limbs softer and more supple, your hair thick and glistening, and your skin glowing due to the extra blood being pumped around your body. You can look glowing and gorgeous, so make yourself feel good with some new pregnancy clothing so you can really enjoy your body as it blooms. Listen to your body and and do what you need to care for yourself. You are doing an extremely important job.

Although you are subtly busy growing a child inside you, you probably still need to continue with daily life as far as possible throughout your pregnancy: work, older children, and other responsibilities. So, what if you're not feeling too well? There are a range of ailments which may affect you including: morning sickness, backache, varicose veins, heartburn, piles and insomnia. What fun!

I list them here so that should you suffer, you know you are not alone, and that it is quite normal for your body to be changing and responding to the fluctuation of hormones and physical changes. This is a time to really listen to your body as these conditions are your body telling you that you need to do something. Consult your doctor or a complementary therapist, and get the help you need. Being open to help is a good skill to develop for motherhood, as is learning to rest when possible.

Here are some suggestions for how to help yourself with some of the more common problems of pregnancy:

Morning sickness: It may be that there isn't much you can do about your morning sickness except to take care of yourself, breathe through it, and let it pass. About 50% of women find it passes at about 14 weeks. Drinking ginger or mint tea can help. Simply put a slice or two of fresh root ginger or a sprig of mint in a mug, top with boiling water and allow to steep then sip gently. You can also use aromatherapy with ginger and mint, or sniff citrus oils such as mandarin, sweet orange or lemon. Eat small meals throughout the day, or if you find a time of day when the sickness clears, eat then. Some women find eating crackers can help. Notice if there are certain activities that make you feel worse and avoid them if possible. I knew I was pregnant with my second baby when I went on a twisty car journey and felt sick. My morning sickness always manifested as car sickness so I tried not to do too much car travel.

Backache: As your body changes shape, so you need to become aware of your changing posture. Larger breasts and a growing belly can change your centre of gravity and curve your back. Make sure you are taking care of your back by keeping it straight and not slouching and just becoming aware of your posture. Pregnancy yoga can really help, as can gentle massage, or warm baths with healing salts.

Varicose veins: These are enlarged veins that can show up in your legs. Drink plenty of water, don't sit or stand in the same position for too long, avoid wearing high heels, and take regular exercise. Massage is not recommended for varicose veins.

Heartburn: When acid from your stomach escapes into the oesophagus due to the increase in progesterone during pregnancy relaxing your stomach valve. Eat at least two hours before going to bed, and take an antacid product which is safe to use during pregnancy.

Piles: Piles can feel lumpy, itchy or sore around your anus and develop due to the extra weight of the baby pushing down on that area. The best thing you can do is avoid them by eating a high fibre diet including plenty of fresh fruit and vegetables. Quinoa has twice as much fibre as other grains and is fantastic as a stool loosener whilst being highly nutritious. Once again regular exercise can save the day too.

Insomnia: I wrote much of this book on insomnia, sitting on the toilet late into the night with notebook and pen, so it's not necessarily a bad thing. If you really are struggling with sleep, try a meditation using an app such as Insight Timer. Yoga Nidra (yoga sleep) is a good way to experience deep relaxation and can give you a sense of having had a good, long sleep, although it takes only 45 minutes. Again this is downloadable from meditation apps or online music stores such as iTunes or Amazon.

Pregnancy is traditionally divided up into three trimesters, or phases, but I include a fourth phase: The first twelve weeks of the baby's life. How we feel during pregnancy is going to be largely dependent on each of us as individuals, but below is a rough guide to each trimester and how you are likely to be feeling. If you have any concerns or worries, make sure you speak to your midwife or doctor.

FIRST TRIMESTER WEEKS 1 – 12

This is the period where mind and body are acclimatizing to your new state. You may feel a tiredness like you've never experienced before, accompanied by an ability to drop off to sleep at any time, anywhere. You may feel sick or nauseous and possibly you're even vomiting ('morning sickness' is a misnomer – it can happen any time). Your sense of smell and taste can become heightened at this time. It's also the time you'll be moving house, doing up a bathroom or some similar stressful household project. (It just seems to be how it goes.) Probably, you haven't told many (if any) people, so along with all the changes happening to your body and emotions, you are carrying a secret laden with feelings of excitement, wonder, amazement, but also maybe fear, confusion, bewilderment and disbelief. You'll have your first scan round about 12 weeks, after which things may start to feel a little more real.

SECOND TRIMESTER WEEKS 13 - 25

It is during this part of the pregnancy that you will probably start to feel better on every level. It's likely that the sickness will have passed and your energy levels should be higher although your body is still extremely busy creating your baby, so you may experience tiredness at times. Your belly will probably be starting to look like a bump and everyone now knows you're pregnant. You may feel like you're starting to settle into your pregnancy and enjoy it. You may begin to feel small kicks and movements from your baby as they become more active. This phase of the pregnancy is sometimes known as 'the honeymoon period' but don't worry if yours is not like that. Every woman, and every pregnancy is different.

THIRD TRIMESTER WEEKS 26 - 40

During the third trimester you will be starting to feel heavier and slower, and by the end you will be desperate to meet your baby and to get your body back! In addition to all the physical changes, your body will be producing a cocktail of hormones that affect your emotions. That, added to the huge change that is imminent, will mean that you really need to be on your own side during this time. You may feel distracted if you are constantly having a conversation with someone who nobody else can see. Isn't it awe inspiring that this miracle of life is happening inside your body? On the other hand, you might just feel like you've been taken over by an alien. Braxton Hicks 'practice' contractions can occur now, when the muscles start tightening in preparation for labour. Later on you may find you are uncomfortable sleeping and that you have vivid dreams. You may feel hotter than usual with the extra blood pumping around your body. Your baby's head will engage some time during these last few weeks, earlier with subsequent babies.

FOURTH TRIMESTER WEEKS 1-12 POST BIRTH

You have had your baby, and you are no longer pregnant, but this is a sensitive and special time in yours and your baby's life. This is a period of discovery: you and your baby discovering each other, yourselves, and your new world. If you are becoming a mother for the first time, you will be feeling quite different from your old, stand alone self. Your baby, too, is experiencing change, from being cosseted in the warm, gentle waters of your womb, to breathing air, and engaging in the outside world of sounds, smells, sights and touch. The first 12 weeks are a whirlwind of feeding, changing, cuddling, crying and sleep deprivation. Your focus shifts with intensity onto this new person for whom you are entirely responsible.

This is such an important time for developing your relationship with your new baby and holding, stroking, talking, singing, and playing with your baby are all pleasures you have anticipated throughout your pregnancy. There is an awful lot to do. It can be tough. But when your baby gives you his or her first smile, you will melt and feel it's all worth it. Take care of yourself during this phase by sleeping when you can, so when your baby does, getting out for some gentle exercise and not expecting too much of yourself. Not getting dressed all day, and having the house in a mess is completely to be expected in this phase. Get help from family and friends so you can concentrate on making a connection with your baby that will develop a nourishing relationship between you as they grow and develop into childhood. There is more about the post-natal period in Chapter 9.

Whilst you are pregnant it is important to be fully aware of what it is you are doing: creating life! You have a little person inside you who is relying on you to care for them. This is a responsibility but also a privilege. Having a baby is not something that's going to happen alongside your usual life. It is going to have a totally life-changing impact, and now, whilst you are pregnant, is a good time to start to think about how you want to bring your baby up, how he or she will fit into your life, how you can give them the best possible care and attention. This is a small human being whose life you have been gifted with. What life gifts do you want to give them?

THINGS TO DO

- ▶ Take some time every day to be with your baby, to sit, breathe deeply, and connect. Rub your belly, envisage what your baby looks like, how she or he feels, and really get to know each other.
- ▶ Start thinking about the kind of mother you would like to be, the kind of parents you and your partner would like to be. This may change when the reality of caring for a baby hits, but it is still useful to have thought through your basic philosophy. Here are a few examples to consider:

Where will your baby sleep: in your bed, in a cot in your room, in a cot in another room?

Pram or sling? Will you be pushing or carrying your baby?

Will you be using childcare? If so, what kind? Grandparents, daycare or a nanny?

Feeding to a schedule or feeding on demand? Breast or bottle?

Chapter Two

NATURAL vs. MEDICAL

"Birth is not an emergency. It is simply an emergence."
Jeannine Parvati Baker

Really what we are calling 'natural' birth is simply a 'normal' birth. Women have been birthing babies for millennia: look at the size of the human race! Medical intervention in industrialised nations became popular from about the 1950's. My dad tells a great story of how as a medical student in the East End of London in the 1960's, he attended a birth as part of his training. He went upstairs to attend to the woman in labour, and stood by watching, astonished as she birthed the baby with no intervention, no equipment, and no noise. In our culture, we have become so accustomed to both the medicalisation of birth, and the drama surrounding it, that we have lost touch with the fact that it really is a normal, daily occurrence.

The creeping caesarean rates give some indication of how far we have come from seeing birth as normal and natural: the highest at over 50% in Turkey, down to 15% in the Netherlands with the US coming in at 32.5% and the UK at 20%.

Roughly 20% of mothers-to-be experience medical complications that necessitate interventions. Problems like eclampsia or placenta previa. Twins or other multiples also require medical intervention, and generally, although not always, the skills for delivering a breech baby (feet first) naturally have been lost amongst birth professionals so this is almost always carried out by caesarian section which is considered safer. In these cases we can be grateful for the medical intervention that keeps both mother and baby alive. About 80% of women should be able to give birth perfectly safely without any medical intervention at all.

In ancient times, across cultures, birthing was the sole preserve of the women of the community. Midwives (the word midwife literally means 'with woman'), mothers and other family members eased the new mother through her birthing process. Since the latter half of the 20th Century childbirth has been treated more and more as a medical problem, rather than a natural process which requires nurturing, support and guidance. Medical birth has removed decisions from the mother, and placed them in the hands of 'expert professionals'.

In addition, the modern medical approach is based on fear. Fear that the mother is not labouring within the right timescales, persistent monitoring to ensure the foetal heart rate is stable, fear of pain, and so on. The hospital environment itself instills fear in the strongest of us. It is anxiety inducing: bright lights, unfamiliar equipment, strangers. It feels threatening as you wonder what they are going to do to you. In the animal kingdom, of which we are a part, mammals seek small, dark places in which to give birth, and they need to feel comfortable and at ease. Imagine an elegant giraffe giving birth, for example, whilst being chased by a lion. It just wouldn't happen. Fear is the very emotion that prevents labour from progressing smoothly. It causes adrenaline to be produced, triggering the 'fight or flight' response, the opposite to the calm, stress reducing hormone, oxytocin which relaxes the body and eases the passage of the baby.

Often the medical approach can trigger what has become known as a 'cascade of intervention'. What this means is that if you start by being induced (see Chapter 8), you are more likely to be given pain relieving drugs, or an epidural and in turn more likely to have a caesarian. So, although birth has come to equal a trip to hospital, there is another way in which to bring a baby into the world, one which can be gentle, peaceful and empowering for the mother-to-be.

By birthing consciously with a deep connection to yourself, and with support, *you* can become the expert on what your needs are during your pregnancy and the birth. By listening closely to yourself, you can guide others towards what you need for your optimum comfort and ease during the birth. A study in Ontario, Canada in 2015 found that for women with low-risk pregnancies, babies delivered at home with a midwife are at no greater risk of harm than those born in hospital with a midwife's assistance.

Imagine your baby easing out, maybe into water, in calm and quiet, a warm bath or shower afterwards, relaxing with your baby son or daughter straight afterwards in your own bed. We are built for birth, women have done it naturally for millennia, and so can you! The next chapter will help you prepare for your birth so you have the greatest opportunity to birth your baby naturally.

There are a number of options open to you for natural birth:

HOME BIRTH USING INDEPENDENT MIDWIVES

The benefit of using an independent midwife as opposed to local midwives is that you have the same midwife or midwives throughout your pregnancy and birth, and can develop a personal relationship. It can really help you relax during labour if you are familiar with, and trust, the people present. Your midwife will visit you during your pregnancy, be present at the birth and support you in the postnatal period. The National Maternity Review (2017) says: 'We found almost total unanimity from mothers that they want their midwife to be with them from the start, through pregnancy, birth and then after birth.'

HOME BIRTH USING NHS MIDWIVES

Did you know that every woman in the UK is entitled to a home birth? In reality, your area may be more or less supportive of it, so your ability to achieve this will be wholly dependent on local policies and procedures. Some may be happy to support a home birth, but not a water birth, and some may be resistant to you having a home birth at all.

HOSPITAL BIRTH

It is possible to have a relatively calm, peaceful and natural birth in a hospital setting. You may feel more relaxed in hospital knowing that medical care is on hand just in case. However, the environment of a hospital can be quite fear inducing with bright lights, equipment and machinery, strangers around you, and this can make the fear response kick in, triggering just the hormones that close your body up, preventing labour from progressing. Also, hospital staff have clinical timeframes in which they expect you to proceed and the chances of intervention are much higher.

You can either visit or take a virtual tour of your local hospital so make your decision based on how you feel about this visit, and whether your wishes will be respected. Make sure what you want is in your birth plan and that you have someone there who can represent your wishes; your partner, a friend, family member, or doula. Your local GP or midwife should be able to give you more information about services in your area.

BIRTH CENTRES

The aim of birth centres is to treat birth as a straightforward, normal thing to happen. Some areas have birth centres, either privately run or NHS. They may be stand-alone, or alongside a hospital. These are units, usually run by midwives, which can have a homely feel to them, and provide medical care whilst allowing you to birth naturally and peacefully in your own way.

'HOME FROM HOME' SUITES IN HOSPITAL

These vary from hospital to hospital, but provide a more 'cosy' environment with private rooms and often with birth pools. Unfortunately, staffing is often an issue, as midwives can be caught up in more 'urgent' cases on the labour ward, but this can prove to be a good halfway compromise between hospital and home.

PRIVATE HOSPITAL

Your ability to give birth naturally in a private hospital will depend entirely on the ethos of that particular hospital. Some private hospitals specialise in highly medicalised births whilst others are excellent with natural births.

THINGS TO DO

- Make your decision about how you would like to birth your baby
- Discuss your thoughts about where you would like to birth with your partner
- Find people to support you in your decision: your partner, your midwife, friends or family
- Research the birthing facilities in your local area

Chapter Three

PREPARE YOURSELF

"Luck is what happens when preparation meets opportunity"
Unknown

Assuming you have now decided that a natural birth is the choice for you, let's talk about preparation. Like any 'labour' be it running in a race or taking an academic test, successfully birthing naturally takes preparation. In fact, preparation is the key to giving yourself the greatest chance to have a natural birth. This can start as soon as you have conceived, or even before. Birth being what it is, it is never totally predictable and sometimes other plans will be in store for you. But, whatever happens, the planning and preparation that will have gone into your natural birth will assist you in remaining calm, healthy and focused regardless of the end result. I start here with a '3 pledge promise' to yourself which I ask you to sign and commit to throughout your pregnancy and beyond.

THE THREE PLEDGE PROMISE OF THE PREGNANT MOTHER

1. I will honour myself and my body whilst I am pregnant, and beyond.

Whilst you are pregnant you are (generally) carrying on with your former life, initially with no outside evidence of any changes. However, inside you will be a maelstrom of different emotions and experiences as you deal with the life coming into being inside you. Not only are you continuing with your life at hand, you are creating another little being.

When you are pregnant you need to pamper yourself and honour yourself more than ever before. I have a 'yummy list' which lists all the treats which make me feel nurtured and warm and gorgeous. I make sure I do at least one of these a day. For example, start the day with meditation or yoga then give yourself an all over body massage followed by a warm shower, put on a few drops of scent and face the day on top of the world. Honour your emotions by acknowledging them, allowing them and being kind to yourself, whatever you may be feeling. All sorts of things come up when you are pregnant. During my final pregnancy I felt extremely frustrated at how slow I became and how I couldn't participate so physically with the other children. However, I had to learn to accept this and bring them along at my pace. Use your pregnancy to build faith in yourself and your body. Indulge yourself in whatever makes you feel good, in body, mind and spirit.

2. I will focus only on positive birth stories.

As soon as anyone knows you are pregnant, they will be desperate to tell you their birth story.

Unfortunately, most of these will be negative. For some reason, it is not usual for people to talk about their positive experiences, unless you really ask. When I was 12 weeks pregnant with my first baby (a very sensitive time) I met up with 3 women who already each had 2 children. I had already decided to have a natural home birth and told them so when they asked where I was having the baby. I was completely ridiculed as they proceeded to tell me all the horrific and gory details of their births in hospital. It was a sorely upsetting experience and I decided there and then to seek out stories of positive births and women who would support my decision. Another friend, shortly after this, lent me her copy of Ina May Gaskin's *'Stories of Childbirth'* and I immersed myself in positive stories of uplifting, inspiring births. So, avoid people who are negative about your choices, or if they are unavoidable, simply do not discuss it with them – take strength in your decision. If anyone does begin to tell you a horror story tell them, thank you, but no, I don't want to hear it. Fill your mind with positive images and talk to others who you think will be positive and supportive too.

3. I will take charge of my birth experience.

The Law of Attraction, simply put, goes like this: in life we get what we focus on. So, focus on misery and negativity, and, guess what, your life will be miserable and negative. Focus on the positive potential and this is where life takes you. Most of all, tune in to the calming 'self' within by stopping, breathing and noticing with mindfulness, what's going on inside. When I say 'I will take charge of my birth experience' I emphasize the 'my'. It is your opportunity to really listen to yourself and what you want, regardless of prevailing culture or what your friends and family believe. It is a major point in your life, where you bring another being into this world through your body, and begin the journey of parenting that child. Consider the birth plan in the Appendix. Add to it. Draw on it. Create it as yours. Then visualise your baby arriving as you have planned. Communicate your plan to your birth partner(s). Most of all enjoy the experience of pregnancy and birth. It may only happen once or only a very few times in your life and you are honoured to be able to do it.

One of the reasons, I believe, why so many women end up having difficult births (aside from medical issues which cannot be avoided) is that they are completely unprepared in a number of areas:

1) Mentally: giving birth is not easy. Having a normal, natural birth requires some effort and thought, some education, and a positive mindset.

2) Emotionally: how do you feel about natural birth? Are you wracked with fear because of your own birth experience. Do you feel under

pressure from friends or family to have medical intervention? Your emotions around your birth will change as your pregnancy progresses, and from pregnancy to pregnancy.

3) Physically: is your body prepared? Do you believe your body can do it? Can you relax?

Let's have a look at these, one by one:

MENTAL PREPARATION

Knowing what is going to happen to you, and to your body will really help you to understand the experience of birth. There are some fantastic birth animations on YouTube which give you a very clear anatomical view of birth, and really helped me to understand how the baby comes out. In our information rich society, knowing and understanding how things happen is so important to our sense of safety. There is more information later in the book about labour, which will help to mentally prepare you for the experience. The second part of your mental preparation is to do with your mindset. Do you believe you can have a natural birth, and are you prepared or preparing for it? Preparing all the practicalities will help: where you want to birth, who with, even down to what you want to wear (if anything), whether you will light candles or have flowers in the room. Attend birth preparation or antenatal classes with your partner or birth partner. In the UK we have the National Childbirth Trust which provides classes for a small fee, and many people make firm family friends at these classes, and tap into a network of local support.

Starting to visualise the birth going as planned will give you great strength and confidence, and also give you the opportunity to deal with any emotions that come up, or any negative voices you may have inside you telling you that you can't do it. This inner critic can pop up at any time of our lives, and learning to deal with it now will have positive repercussions throughout your life. The first step in dispelling the inner critic is to recognise it. Once you see it for what it is, a negative voice picked up from past experiences, family, friends, and your own beliefs, you can see it as something outside yourself, something you can observe, and dismiss. Meditation is a great tool to recognise the inner critic, and still it, and combining this with a birth visualisation is a powerful way to start to create the birth you would love. At the same time as dismissing the inner critic, this is your time to work on your PMA (Positive Mental Attitude). 'Yay! I can do it!' This is so important that I have created an entire chapter, Chapter 5, covering PMA in greater depth.

EMOTIONAL

During pregnancy you may find yourself in a more heightened emotional state than usual due to the cocktail of hormones coursing through your body. That's fine. In fact, it's useful to be aware of your emotions in relation to your birth because your emotional state and the physical state of your body are intrinsically linked. Whatever you feel emotionally impacts on your body. Have you ever found that when you have been going through a tough time emotionally, or been feeling a bit down, this is when you may get a cold or other illness? Or after exercise, the relationship works in reverse: your body feels great, so your emotions are lifted. This is not a case of dismissing all negative emotions. That would be impossible. It is about becoming aware of them, of allowing them to be, noticing they are there, and maybe exploring them through talking with a supportive friend or family member, your midwife, or even a counselor or therapist, if you feel you need professional help.

In the last month of pregnancy with my last child, I felt such fear about the birth. I climbed into the warm water of the birth pool, wallowing in the soothing waters. My husband stood at my side and I said to him, "I'm scared." I felt it, I really felt it: tears welling up, a feeling of hopelessness, like I just couldn't do it this time. He listened, and just in the act of allowing that emotion room to express itself, the fear and hopelessness dissipated. Fear is a common emotion relating to giving birth, and unsurprisingly so. We are going through a challenging physical experience that we have not done before.

Other emotions may arise that are triggered by the birth, but related to past traumas or experiences, and your birth experience is an opportunity to explore those. Get yourself a journal and write freely about your emotions to get them out of your head and onto paper. Or you can create artwork to express yourself: painting or drawing your way through. The Birth Art Cafe in Hertfordshire in the UK specifically uses art to support women with birth, and the Birthing from Within system also advocates the use of art to deal with the inner experience of birth.

PHYSICAL

Several words spring to mind when I think about the physical state required for giving birth: strong, open, soft, relaxed, surrendered. The tight, taut muscles we cultivate through intense physical exercise help with strength, but not with softness. Learning to relax is another skill that we need to learn to deal with our everyday life of busy schedules and to-do lists. Again this is how the physical interacts with the mental and emotional. If you are caught up in emotional or mental stress this will be expressed in your body. The best way to create the physical state you need for birth is by practicing yoga. Find a local pregnancy yoga class, or have a go at some of the exercises below. Joining a class will also give you great emotional support and friendship which is invaluable during your pregnancy. You will find some like minded mamas to be who will support your natural birth plan. I made my closest bunch of mama friends through pregnancy yoga as we laughed, cried, relaxed and chatted through our classes.

SOME SIMPLE YOGA POSES

Always do yoga on an empty stomach, at least 2 hours after food. First thing in the morning is an excellent time to practice, or last thing at night before you go to bed. Aim to practice every day, but be happy if you've managed three times in a week! You don't need any special clothes, so long as they are comfortable and offer you free movement. Have a blanket or wrap on hand.

Sit on the floor with your legs crossed, your spine straight, your shoulders relaxed and your chin very gently tucked in. Place your hands on you knees, palms up, and gently touch the thumb and forefinger together, if this feels comfortable. Close your eyes. Breathe three or more long, slow breaths, and, becoming still prepare yourself to be fully present for the postures. You will notice your mind being very active, and this is normal. Every time your mind wanders, gently bring your attention back to noticing the breath as it enters and leaves through your nose.

This sequence is simple and gentle and will start to create the supple joints and openness you need for birth. It is essential in yoga to combine physical movement with breath, and it is this breath awareness that will really help you as you progress through your pregnancy, and into labour and birth.

1) Still sitting in cross legged position, begin making slow, small circles with your torso, moving from your hips. Coordinate the breath with the movement, breathing in as you come forward, and out as you go back. Start in a clockwise direction, gradually making the circles bigger. Make about 20 circles, making them smaller again until you come back to centre. Take a deep breath here, then repeat the practice anti clockwise. **Take a few deep, relaxing breaths.**

2) Holding the ankles, gently begin to flex the spine, breathing in as you arch your chest open, and out as you arch your chest inwards. Think of this as your spine flexing and keep your shoulders still. Move your hands to your knees and repeat. **Take a few deep, relaxing breaths.**

3) Breathing in, shrug your shoulders up to your ears, breathing out, let them gently release. Do this ten times or so, then squeeze your

shoulders up to your ears, and drop them down with a big sigh. **Take a few deep, relaxing breaths.**

4) Neck exercises: Breathing in tip your head left, towards your shoulder, breathe out as you gently tip your head the other way. Repeat three times. Next, left to right, breathing in left, breathing out right, again three times. Finally, rotate your head in circles, three times clockwise, three times anti-clockwise. Come to centre and yes… **Take a few deep, relaxing breaths.**

THINGS TO DO

- Sign and commit to your Three Pledge Promise at the end of the book
- Draw up a 'yummy list' and enjoy!
- Start thinking about your ideal birth experience
- Use the Birth Meditation and Visualisation once a day
- Attend a pregnancy yoga class

Chapter Four

LOOKING AFTER NO. 1

"We cannot nurture others from a dry well. We need to take care of our own needs first, then we can give from our surplus, our abundance.'
Jennifer Louden

Use your pregnancy to build faith in your body, mind and spirit. Weekly treatments during pregnancy are not a luxury, but a necessity. Your hard-working organs and muscles get a chance to rejuvenate with an hour on the massage table. If it is too costly for you, find a student who needs a practice patient, or ask your partner to help out. Self-massage can also be extremely relaxing and effective. Massage your body from head to toe with sweet almond oil before you have a shower in the morning. Your skin will glow and it will assist your joints, your internal organs, and your general feeling of well-being. (Do consult a qualified practitioner about suitable aromatherapy oils as some are contraindicated in pregnancy). Below are further suggestions of how to look after yourself during pregnancy, and beyond.

REFLEXOLOGY

This can be even more relaxing than a massage as you don't have to move, or take your clothes off, and can easily switch off your brain whilst the therapist works on pressure points in your feet. A good therapist can tell where you may have problems, for example if you need to drink more fluids, or have tension which can prevent problems from becoming more serious. It can be good for foetal positioning later on, encouraging the baby into a good position for the birth, and to bring labour on if you are overdue. It is incredibly relaxing and beneficial throughout pregnancy (and afterwards).

YOGA

This is the best way to keep your body in optimum condition during pregnancy and to prepare for birth. Once you have been guided by a class, you can tailor a practice at home to suit your own needs day by day. There are pregnancy yoga or birth preparation yoga classes in most areas. Look for the Janet Balaskas trained Active Birth Yoga teachers or find other classes local to you. They will not only relax and support you through pregnancy but may be a source of your first friendships as a mother, as you share this magnificent time together. Half an hour of practice at home every day will keep your body moving and relieve aches, pains and stiffness. Light a candle, tune in, limber up, and connect with your baby. Bliss!

REST

The fact is, you will probably be more tired. So, the greatest tonic is to rest and lie down whenever you can. You may be legally entitled to time off work for pregnancy related classes, appointments or rest if you need it. Accept that you will need to slow down – even while you are lying down, your body is still actively engaged in the complicated process of forming a new life. If friends or family come to visit, learn to accept help and to take the opportunity to lie down or have them look after other children for you. This is something I found extremely hard to accomplish as it is not natural in our culture (or in my nature) to accept help, and resting, or stillness is not generally valued. However, by my fourth pregnancy I was quite expert at letting others step in, and any offers were gratefully received.

HEALTHY EATING

I'm not going to patronise you by telling you what to eat. Suffice to say, eat healthily and try not to overeat. You do need some extra calories to support the baby – estimates range from between 200 to 500 calories per day, depending on the stage of pregnancy. Grantly Dick-Read points out in his seminal book, 'Childbirth without Fear' that women can be healthy in pregnancy from a wide variety of culturally appropriate diets. Vegetarianism/veganism is also ok so long as you approach with awareness and understanding of the nutrients required.

HEALTHY LIFESTYLE

In our modern world we are surrounded by toxins – in the air we breathe, the products we use and the food we eat. Pregnancy is a great time to consider what we are putting on, in and around our bodies, and to think about how this is going to affect our choice of products for our new babies. The main chemicals to avoid in body and cleaning products are sodium laurel (or laureth) sulphate and propylene glycol. In order to avoid as many toxins as possible and keep your body as healthy as possible for the long haul, consider the following:

1. Eat organic: easily available by delivery eg. Able & Cole, Riverford, or grow your own.
2. Use gentle, non-toxic, bath and cosmetic products. Available from your health store. Deodorant is a particular one to mention as regular deodorants can cause blockages in the pores leading to underarm lumps which can affect the breasts. Try a crystal deodorant. I swear by mine. Tisserand, Organic Surge and Faith in Nature products are all good, but there is a wealth of products out there if you look for them.

3. Household cleaning products: use natural products such as lemon juice, bicarbonate of soda or white vinegar, or alternative products which have none of the harmful ingredients, also available from health stores or online

SWIMMING

Swimming gently exercises every muscle in the body so is perfect for pregnancy. It is lovely towards the end of pregnancy when the water supports the expanding weight of your bump.

WALKING

Walking is another excellent way to keep active and rested, although due to the looseness of the ligaments it is generally thought that walking on uneven ground should not be recommended.

OTHER EXERCISE

Most exercise is fine to continue throughout pregnancy if you are already doing it, for example cycling and running. This is not a good time to take up a new exercise though. Consider the risks of activities such as horse-riding and skiing as a fall could hurt your baby.

WHAT SUSTAINS YOU?

Personally, I don't feel myself if I haven't got a good book on the go, I need time with female friends, I need to write, I need time in nature and to knit, to name a few. What do you need to make you feel sustained, supported and like you? This is an essential skill to develop for when you have your children as well. Pregnancy can be a time of introspection, of thinking about what is important to you, and of renewed focus, so this is a good opportunity to really consider what makes you joyful and love your life.

MEDICAL TREATMENTS

Consider natural and complementary therapies whilst you are pregnant so as not to introduce potentially harmful drugs into yours and the baby's bloodstream.

Homeopathy - available from many local pharmacists or seek a qualified homeopath

Bach Flower or Australian Flower essences

Raspberry Leaf Tea, contrary to popular belief can be taken throughout pregnancy to tone the uterus. Also available in capsule form.

PERINEAL MASSAGE

As you know, this is the part of you between vagina and anus (sometimes called the taint). This part of your body has to stretch during birth so making it supple by massaging with some wheatgerm oil (or other very rich massage oil, preferably with high vitamin E content) can help to soften up the area in preparation for birth

THINGS TO DO

- ▶ What sustains you? What makes you feel great? Take some time to think about the things that make you really feel good. Write them down and indulge in them wherever possible, at least daily.
- ▶ Book yourself in for a treatment.
- ▶ Reassess how healthy your lifestyle is in light of your pregnancy. Can you improve it?

Chapter Five

PMA: POSITIVE MENTAL ATTITUDE

> "If you intend to be of assistance, your eye is not upon the trouble but upon the assistance, and that is quite different. When you are looking for a solution, you are feeling positive emotion— but when you are looking at a problem, you are feeling negative emotion."
>
> **Abraham**

In simple terms, in life, you reap what you sow. If you sow seeds of doubt and fear, be sure to double them on the way back to you. If however, you sow seeds of joy and light, wellness and health, these will return to you in abundance. This takes constant vigilance, but is well worth the effort. During my fourth pregnancy I went through a phase of feeling very uncomfortable and unable to sleep. For about 2 weeks, I focused on the problem of my discomfort and how tired I was and became ever more grumpy. Then, I awoke to the fact that by focusing on my discomfort, I wasn't allowing myself to find a solution to it. As soon as I started to focus on solutions (for example ensuring I did some yoga stretches every day) to becoming more comfortable, my body began to relax and I felt much, much better. Positive mental attitude (PMA) will get you through pregnancy, birth, and life itself!

Another way to greatly enhance your positive attitude is through the use of affirmations. Affirmations are positively phrased statements. They can be used to convince the subconscious mind of something of which the conscious mind can be a little sceptical! Repeat them daily. Put them up on your fridge or bathroom mirror. Eventually you will believe in what they say. Their power is infinite. Choose one or more of the below to focus on your birth, or make up one of your own.

"I am getting all the sleep I need to feel relaxed and vibrant."

"I am looking after my body and my baby in every way."

"I am enjoying regular rests."

"I feel totally calm about the whole birth experience."

"My body is totally capable of birthing my baby."

"I am completely relaxed and calm about my birth."

"My baby will be born peacefully and naturally into water."

"My baby will be born peacefully and naturally at home."

"My body is perfectly designed to birth my baby."

"I am strong and capable."

THINGS TO DO

Write yourself an affirmation.

Think about the issue that is most bugging you about your birth, and write yourself an affirmation. If, for example, it is that your birth canal is too small, reverse that worry and write, "my birth canal is the perfect size to birth my baby". Do you get it?

Chapter Six

LOOKING AFTER NO. 2 (THE MAN IN YOUR LIFE)

"You've got to look after your man, because at the end of it all, the children leave home, and you're left with him."

Grandma Nita and Great Auntie Freda

When the test result showed positive for my first baby, my husband blanched. He looked absolutely terrified. Although you are the one visibly going through the emotional and physical strains of a pregnancy, your husband or partner will be with you all the way, having his own emotional reaction to your changing physicality, the new life inside you that is part of him, and the change in role that will be demanded of him later. He may not know how to express this and may instead start to worry about you excessively, spend lots more time at work, or start drinking and spending more time with his mates. But, hopefully not…

He may be in awe of your impending motherhood, and he is almost certainly terrified for you for the birth. Your job is to guide him through the process and communicate your needs along the way. Many men are scared about natural births as they don't want to see their wives or partners in pain. They are scared about home births because they worry that they will have to deliver the baby. (Note: men never deliver babies. They always come from a woman's body). My husband was totally resistant to a home birth at first. Like most people, he had only heard awful stories about birth, and felt it was a medical issue. He was reassured, however, when he met our midwife. By birth three and four, the midwife didn't make it, and he and I were the only ones present. He coped admirably and both babies came safely and calmly into the world.

There are a number of things to remember about men, which will come in very handy for your pregnancy, birth, and in your newly establishing relationship later:

1. They really like to be appreciated and praised. Specific, descriptive praise is the best such as, 'That was brilliant of you to think about doing the washing-up. I really appreciated it!'

2. You have to be really direct and say exactly what you want. They are decidedly bad at guessing that the harrumphing and eye-rolling mean you really need a break and could he cook dinner tonight.

3. They like to know what's in it for them, for example, if he does the washing up, it will give you time together later.

This is your opportunity to spend time together, develop and strengthen your relationship, and do all the things it will be much trickier to do when you are parents of a small baby.

So, do you involve your man in the appointments? Does he attend the birth? How involved do you or he want him to be? Until the latter part of the twentieth century, fathers-to-be were not involved in the birth at all. These days it is expected that the father will be present but not all men are cut out for it, or want to be there. Birth really is women's stuff, and although it could be considered an honour to be present at the birth, not all dads want to. (In a recent interview in Juno Magazine, Michel Odent, the French pioneer of water birth, suggests that it's possible that having a man present at the birth can actually slow down labour, whether it be the father, or even a medical professional.) Discuss it with him, and make sure you make the right decision between you. In addition, if you think you'd feel more comfortable without him there, that's fine too. Having said that, it's the most wonderful experience to share together, and having a slightly loved-up feeling between you can help the baby to come out.

THINGS TO DO

Have an evening in together.

Treat yourself to a cosy evening in together, no distractions. Prepare a delicious dinner. Talk openly and frankly about the birth and the baby, no raised eyebrows, just no-judgements listening. Make your evening together a regular, say weekly, event. It's a great habit to get into for when your baby is born and time together becomes more scarce.

Chapter Seven

THIS IS IT! LABOUR AND BIRTH

"We have a secret in our culture, it's not that birth is painful, it's that women are strong."

Laura Stavoe Harm

As I believe I have already mentioned, birth is the most natural thing in the world. We women are built for it, and are honoured to be the ones to do it. To give you faith in your body, I am going to give you a short lesson in anatomy. The illustration below shows the female pelvis.

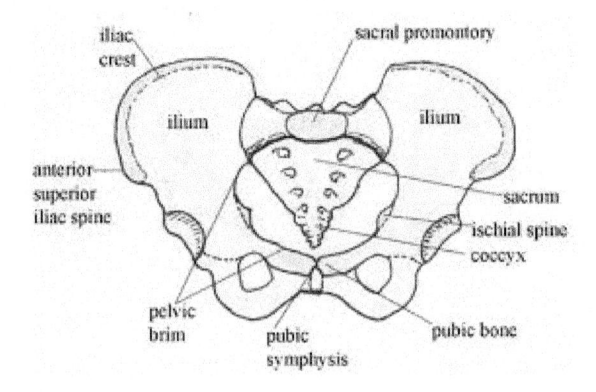

There are two most important things to draw from this illustration:

1. The size of the pelvis. This part of our anatomy is the perfect size for a baby to come through. If you don't believe me, measure for yourself (see Things To Do below for how to do this).

2. The coccyx, at the base of the spine has to ease backwards and open out in order for the baby to slide out. It is obvious to see that if there is pressure on this area, for example if you are lying down, the coccyx cannot open and the aperture for the baby will be much smaller. The conclusion to draw from this is to remain upright during labour. Add to this the force of gravity, and it's a no-brainer.

I was recently watching a programme on TV about teenage pregnancy. Television, in general, horribly misrepresents the birth experience, and, as ever, this one had me shouting at the telly. The mother-to-be was in her 17th hour of labour with her mother, sister, and boyfriend (still with his coat on) in the room, a midwife prodding around downstairs, and, this is what I find absolutely inconceivable – she was lying down! To me, this just seems like the most basic of errors, the most simple of mechanical problems which could have been solved, and ended the young woman's trial with a bit of walking around and remaining upright. I don't understand how a midwife can be present and fail to recognise a basic fact of human anatomy which could have led to a much more positive outcome.

Before I continue about labour and the birth itself, I want to tell you a little about the due date, which you will probably have been given early on in your pregnancy. Please be aware that this is a fairly random date based on an average gestation period. It is generally accepted that babies can healthily arrive anywhere between 37 and 42 weeks. Just an aside, but interesting anyway – in France the gestational period is calculated as 41 weeks. If you are being pressured into hospital for an induction, bear this in mind. You may have more time than the medical services would have you believe.

LABOUR

It is easy to consider labour as having started when you feel the first twinge, which is why so many women report a 3 day labour. My midwife suggests that you're not in real labour until the point where you can no longer talk on the phone! This isn't a particularly scientific indication, and may not be true in all cases. The standard onset of labour is described as strong regular contractions lasting at least sixty seconds occurring every three minutes and being three to four cms dilated. There is evidence to say true labour may be considered to start at 6cm. I would say it is when you are at a point of no return as it were. If the flow of oxytocin stops, labour will halt even when a woman is fully dilated. It isn't possible to will yourself into labour however nature definitely allows you to halt labour if the conditions aren't right. Some women birth babies with shorter contractions and some with less frequent contractions. Labour is unique with each woman and every baby.

Labour is when your body starts to ease the baby out into the world. It does this via an interchange of hormones between the baby's body and your own. It is triggered by a hormonal change in the baby which says, "I'm ready!" and then causes a chain of reactions in your body which will bring your baby through the birth canal. The main thing that happens is that your uterus contracts whilst your cervix dilates. The cervix is like the gateway to the birth canal, and the bit that is referred to when you hear people saying they were '5 centimetres' etc. I've never been measured or even touched in that area during a birth. My midwife assures me there are other, less intrusive signs as to how far a labour is progressing, and I don't know about you, but I'm rather averse to having unnecessary hands up my vagina.

So, back to the plot: labour is when you are traditionally said to be having 'contractions'. Now, although, as I have described, this is factually correct in terms of the uterus action, I feel it is a misnomer in terms of what is the crux of the matter – the cervix, which is, rather than contracting, opening. So, call me picky, but I find it much more helpful to think of them as 'openings' (In 'Spiritual Midwifery' Ina May Gaskin calls them 'rushes'). So, when I'm in labour, I am then grateful for each opening and imagining openness and space through which my baby will come.

1. THE ONSET OF LABOUR

There are a number of different ways to tell if labour has started, and your baby is imminent. You may have a 'show', where some of the plug of blood and mucous from your cervix comes away, and you'll find blood in your underwear. You may start to feel tightenings or pains across your belly, or your waters may break, resulting in a feeling that you have wet yourself. On the other hand, none of these things are necessarily guarantees that labour has commenced. Even for my fourth baby, I wasn't quite sure that he was coming, and the midwife came out a week before he was born as I was sure my labour had started. So, although you may have some indications that the baby is coming, you may not know that you are actually in labour until you feel the powerful sensations across your belly that leave you in no doubt.

2. THE STAGES OF LABOUR

Labour is traditionally divided up into three sections. The first stage is the stage where your body begins to open up, your cervix to dilate, and your baby to get into position. Then there is the bit called 'transition'. This is a phase where often nothing very much happens at all, and it can be quite frustrating, as you felt you were nearing the birth, and then suddenly, everything stops. Not every woman experiences transition. During the second stage, you will get 'pushy' sensations which can be extremely intense, but probably won't last long as the baby is on its way! If you are upright, and everything is progressing fine, this is the time to follow your instincts and allow your body to push the baby out. It has been at this point in each of my births that I felt I was losing it, and had to take some seriously deep breaths, and tell myself to get a grip.

Next is the exciting bit of the second stage, the bit when your baby is born: the moment everyone has been waiting for, and the moment you have been gearing yourself towards for the past 9 months. First, the baby's head crowns. You can reach down and feel the head between your legs.

Shortly after this the head will be born, facing towards your back. That's the hard bit over with, the head being the largest part. Shortly after the head, the baby's body turns through 45°, and the shoulders slip through the birth canal, followed inevitably by the body. And that's it. Your baby is born. In fact, disregarding labour, the actual birthing of the baby lasts moments. Blink and you'll miss it, which is why I'm such an advocate of preserving your awareness during this supremely precious moment. This is what you've been waiting for! Breathe deeply, and allow your baby to slip from your body. Be gentle on yourself and your baby, trust, and enjoy! But, what about pushing? Your body will push your baby out from the inside, and you will feel some 'pushy' sensations, but whether you actually need to push or not will depend on how your labour has progressed and how open your body is. You will be able to depend on your midwife or doula to guide you here.

Finally, once you think it's all over, you still have the placenta to birth. This is the third stage of labour. Bringing the baby to your breast for a feed stimulates the uterus to contract, and to expel the placenta. It may take half an hour or so for it to be delivered.

PAIN – DOES IT HURT?

I would be lying if I said it didn't hurt. However, there are a number of qualifying conditions that come with this pain that make it different from any other pain you will have experienced. Firstly, you get your baby at the end of it, so the motivation to get through it is immense, like a marathon runner who has been training for months. Secondly, it is not usually constant. You'll have a contraction, then it goes away and you can rest. Thirdly, the moment of birth is exactly that – a moment, and yes, it does hurt, but have you ever burnt yourself? Have you ever fallen over and hurt yourself? The answers are probably yes, but it only lasted a moment, and then you were fine. Fourthly, by being relaxed, at ease and totally surrendering to the experience, you can minimise the pain. Pain is enhanced by fear, so if you can deal with any fears you have beforehand,

and create the optimum conditions for a loving and peaceful birth, the pain will be much minimised. It's not wrong to feel fearful. In fact it's quite natural. Even with my fourth baby, I was wallowing in the birth pool a few days before his birth and talking to my husband about how scared I was about it. It really helps to voice your fears, and face them. And finally, pain is an experience not just of the body, but of the mind. If you can get your mind under control, breathe, and keep your focus on being relaxed and enjoying the experience, then you're laughing all the way to the delivery.

"…if a person's basic state of mind is serene and calm, then it is possible for this inner peace to overwhelm a painful physical experience." His Holiness the Dalai Lama

PAIN AS A RITE OF PASSAGE?

Rites of passage are found when a person transitions from one social state to another. It may be worth thinking about the pain of childbirth as a rite of passage into motherhood. It certainly focuses you on the importance of your impending role as a mother, and the enormity of what you are doing by bringing a life into this world. It makes it a memorable and intense experience, and it marks you out as a survivor highlighting qualities such as strength and endurance, the ability to weather a storm and stillness in the face of adversity: qualities which will be so useful in your ongoing journey as a mother.

WHAT'S IT REALLY LIKE?

I was chatting about this to another mother of four, and what she said was, 'no-one really tells you that it's just like doing a great big poo'. So, there you go, unromantic as it is, it's just like doing a great big poo. Except what comes out the other end is far prettier.

WHAT YOU CAN DO TO MAKE IT EASIER AND MORE FUN...
1. HIRE AN INDEPENDENT MIDWIFE/DOULA

When I asked my midwife, after several visits, exactly what her role would be at the birth, and what she would actually do, she told me she would sit in the corner and drink coffee. Now this was a rather modest assessment as she was able to comfort me in the more tricky moments, give information, massage the right spots, check the baby's heart rate, generally watch for problems and probably a thousand other things that she was incredibly subtle about. However, the point she was trying to make was that she would be as unobtrusive as possible. Her role, and that of a doula, is to be there with you, to support you and to inspire you with confidence to be able to birth your baby. The difference between the two? A midwife is medically qualified and a doula offers practical and emotional support, but not medical.

2. CHILL!

The hormones that got the baby in there are the same ones that will get it out. Known as 'the love hormone', oxytocin is excreted when you are relaxed and turned on. It is the same hormone that helps to send the right messages to your body, and to your baby, about opening and relaxing. (It is counteracted by feelings of fear which encourage the hormone adrenalin which in turn stimulates the 'fight or flight' reflex and makes your body tighten and contract in preparation for its aggressor.)

This is the most important aid to a natural birth. If you are relaxed and at ease, the baby should slip out easily. This can be achieved through your environment, the people present and most importantly your attitude towards the whole experience. Especially ensure that your shoulders are relaxed, and your mouth and jaw area, which are said to be energetically connected to the cervix. So relaxed mouth equals relaxed cervix. Laugh, have fun, and you won't even know you're in labour!

During labour with my second baby, the midwives sat in our living room (drinking their coffee) and we all chatted and joked as I occasionally leant over some furniture for deep breathing. I was gobsmacked when something my midwife had noticed triggered her to suggest I 'head on up to the birth pool if you want to use it'. I didn't even realise the baby was imminent.

Most importantly, remember to b r e a t h e… Learning to control the breath is essential. By this, I don't mean learning complicated breathing techniques, puffing, panting or specific breaths for specific bits of labour. All you need to do is learn how to do long, deep breathing, and then use it during your labour and birth. A yoga or meditation class can help with this. Or simply try this: sit on the floor, cross-legged with a cushion underneath you if you need to, or if you're more comfortable, sit on a chair. Keep your spine straight and active. Close your eyes. Feel your breath expand into your lower belly, upper belly, chest, and all the way to your upper chest. Then slowly exhale in reverse. Equalise the breath, and make sure you're not holding it. Begin by counting to four on the in breath, then four on the out breath. After a few breaths, gradually increase your count. Do this for 11 minutes. Do it regularly in the run up to your birth, and see how calm and reassured it makes you feel.

3. HAVE A WATER BIRTH

Water can be a great source of comfort, relaxation and pain relief during labour, as well as a gentle way to welcome your baby into the world.

WHAT DO YOU NEED?

Firstly, decide on a pool. Do you want to hire or buy, want wood, plastic, heated or unheated? Ultimately, it's your decision and will depend on your budget and wishes. I always had a wood-sided pool with a filter and heater so it could be ready beforehand. It is no longer recommended to have a pre heated pool, in fact it is considered very risky. You need to run fresh warm water for the labour. If using a static pool that is plumbed in it needs to be thoroughly cleaned. If using an inflatable pool a new liner must be used for the birth although of course you can use the pool without a liner or another liner during the antenatal period. It needs to be at body temperature for optimum conditions.

Secondly, you'll need a sieve – yes it's true! With all the letting go and opening of your body, it's likely there will be some poo. Don't worry, though, it's the kind of thing that will pass you by as you concentrate on bigger things.

Thirdly, you'll need a bath mat for climbing out onto, and plenty of towels to wrap you and your newborn baby in.

WHERE DO YOU PUT IT?

People are often unsure where to site a birth pool, and there are stories floating around about the pool and contents crashing their way through first floor ceilings. As far as I am aware, these rumours are unfounded. The space needs to be able to take the weight of 8 adults standing close together. My pools have always been on a first floor, and no mishaps of that nature have occurred. The main thing is that the pool needs to be sited near a tap (this usually means near kitchen or bathroom) and near an electricity socket if you're going to have a pump. It's preferable to have a small, secluded space, or at least somewhere you will feel safe.

WHEN SHOULD YOU GET THE POOL, WHEN SHOULD YOU FILL IT UP AND WHEN SHOULD YOU GET IN?

For hygiene and safety reasons it is recommended that the pool is filled as near as possible to the time you are going to get in. Although it can be lovely to fill it before the birth and have a wallow, you will need to empty it and refill it for the birth itself. Older children will love it!' When you get in the pool during your labour or birth will be entirely up to you and your midwife and/or doula. There are various recommendations about when is the optimum time to get in the pool in order not to slow the labour, but I defer to the professionals in this. You may want to labour in the pool and get out to deliver, or you may feel you want to remain in the pool for the birth itself. It will all depend on how you feel on the day.

WHO SHOULD BUILD AND FILL THE POOL? WHO WILL CLEAN IT AFTERWARDS?

Building the pool is a great way for husbands/partners to feel involved and useful during the whole process. Alternatively, for a few more pennies, some pool companies will do it. The cleaning afterwards, likewise, must be delegated. This is a little more sensitive as there will be bodily fluids, including some blood, so just be aware of that. If you have a doula, or independent midwife, they may be able to help.

WHY HAVE A WATER BIRTH?

Water birth was pioneered by French obstetrician, Michel Odent in the early 1970's. Water birth is now a common and accepted method of giving birth. His philosophy is all about helping the mother work with her body, rather than against it.

A water birth will be for you if you love water! If you find it soothing, calming, restful and restorative, a water birth is for you. If you are not a water person, don't have a water birth, however much it seems the thing to do. There are other, drier ways to have a calm and peaceful birth experience that are for you.

The benefits of a water birth are as much the benefits of a home birth: bringing your baby into the world in a peaceful, homely setting that is comforting for the whole family and allowing you full movement to find your own comfortable positions. The added benefits of water are the pain relief, the comfort of the water taking your weight, and the gentle passage of the baby into the world.

4. HYPNOBIRTHING

Also known as the Mongan Method, this technique uses self-hypnosis, relaxation and breathing techniques which you can learn through audio format, or classes. Hypnobirthing encourages you to have a natural, enjoyable birth experience through antenatal education. I don't have any direct experience of it, but there is plenty of information on the hypnobirthing website where you can find a practitioner or classes.

5. ENVIRONMENT

Human beings are mammals. Mammals like to give birth in seclusion, calmly, peacefully and quietly without the stressors of other animals (people) being present or other scary things. The hormones responsible for delivering the baby work much better under these conditions. Create a calm environment, and only have people there who you are absolutely sure you want to be there (preferably with their coats off). Smooching with your partner can help those hormones too. The same hormones which got the baby in there can actually help to get it out too.

6. ENERGY LEVELS

Labour is as it suggests, 'work', so you will need plenty of energy to keep going. Make sure you eat when you are still able to, and have drinks available throughout your labour. If you like sugary drinks, or juice, these can help to keep your energies up. Water is good too.

7. SILLY WALKS

These are taken from Dr. Gowri Motha's 'Gentle Birth Method" and are inspired by Dr Francoise Freedman, creator of Birthlight yoga. They add to the topic of keeping upright and I'm sure these walks and wiggles sped up my labours no end. Even if they didn't, they kept us laughing, which is useful as well. It is helpful to practice them throughout your pregnancy.

Charlie Chaplin walking: Put your feet out at an angle. Now shuffle around whilst wiggling the hips and imagine your baby coming down into the pelvic cavity.

Elephant walk: Walk forward with giant steps, lifting your knee up and out to the side. This helps to open the pelvis.

Camel Walk: Lift your foot up high and as you bring them down, scoop your pelvis forward and make a circular motion with your pelvis and belly. Looks strange, but great for the lower back.

AFTER THE BIRTH

Your midwife will do an APGAR test which is a simple assessment of how the baby is doing at birth. The APGAR score is an ongoing assessment of the baby in real time at birth up to ten minutes later. If the score is low the midwife will need to act to assist the baby with breathing or circulation. It is recorded at one minute, five minutes and ten minutes to have a record of the assessment made, and changes in the baby's condition. This can be done with your babe in arms. You really don't have to do anything for a little while. Be still and welcome the baby to your bare skin. Skin to skin contact immediately after birth has been shown to have a number of beneficial effects in helping the baby to thrive, particularly if they are small or premature. Offer your baby the breast, cuddle for a while, as you take in the experience. The umbilical cord will then need to be cut – a great job for dads (if they want to), or you can do it yourself, or leave it up to the midwife. Whoever does it, wait until it has stopped pulsing and the baby has obtained the last drops of nutrients from it. (Lotus birth is when you leave the placenta attached until the cord drops off naturally. This can take about two weeks.) The midwife will then check the placenta is intact and if you're interested, show you this amazing organ that's kept your baby alive.

OTHER USEFUL TOOLS FOR A NATURAL LABOUR

Yoga calms and opens the body. As labour begins, consider sitting and doing a few yoga poses or breathing exercises to still and ground yourself.

Walking up stairs opens the pelvis, especially if done two at a time, but don't overdo it and tire yourself out.

Tens machine – can help, can be a distraction. Sends pain-limiting electrical impulses to the brain.

Homeopathy – Helios do a kit especially for pregnancy and birth. You can self-prescribe, or get your birth partner/midwife involved

Massage – You'll know at the time if this is helpful or not and where it should be applied (As I said to my husband, "Massage my back, lower lower, ah just there! Aagh, get off!")

THINGS TO DO

Measure your pelvis.

You will need a piece of paper, a pen, and a soft tape measure.

Squat down. Now feel the bone at the front of your pubis and place the tape measure there. Then take the tape measure to the bone at the base of your spine (the coccyx). Plot these measurements on your paper. Then do the same with the side-to-side bones, from one side of the pelvis to the other, and plot these on your paper. Now, loosely join up the four points to make a rough circle. This indicates the size of your opening – perfect for a baby's head!

LABOUR HINTS SUMMARISED

- ▶ Keep upright/keep moving
- ▶ Instil the atmosphere with calm
- ▶ Breathe

- Let it happen
- Trust in yourself

Chapter Eight

JUST IN CASE – MEDICAL INFORMATION AND TERMINOLOGY

"Forewarned is forearmed"
Ancient proverb

Although I sincerely hope that you do not require medical attention, sometimes it just happens, and you are going to have a much more pleasant experience of it if you know what's going on. So, here's some stuff from the medics to help you understand some of the terms:

INDUCTION

Induction means the use of medical intervention to bring on labour. The medical professionals seem quite keen to intervene and bring the baby on, rather than waiting for nature to take its course. You should be kept an eye on if you are two weeks or more overdue, or if meconium is found in your waters. (Meconium is the first poo your baby expels, full of red blood cells, very dark in colour, and sticky).

MEMBRANE SWEEP

This is a procedure performed by your midwife or doctor to try to bring the baby on. They will sweep a finger round the cervix to disturb the membranes attaching the baby, and this stimulates the production of prostglandins which stimulate the baby to be born. It can be offered at 40 weeks.

ARTIFICIAL RUPTURE OF THE MEMBRANES (ARM)

The amniotic sac is broken with a knitting needle type device (ARM, or artificial rupture of the membranes)

OXYTOCIN INDUCED LABOUR

A drip containing a synthetic version of the hormone oxytocin stimulates the body to begin labour, which can be more intense and painful than a natural delivery, though not always.

GAS & AIR

Also known as Entonox, this is actually an odourless concoction of nitrous dioxide and oxygen which can make you feel heady, a bit sick, giggly and can take the edge off the pain.

PETHIDINE

A synthetic version of morphine used for pain relief. Can make the baby sleepy post delivery.

EPIDURAL

In a low dose, known as ambulatory epidural, as you can walk around, although women often report that this is not the case. An epidural is when an anaesthetic is injected into your spine, to cause numbness to your lower body.

ASSISTED BIRTH

All assisted techniques require you to be lying down, and are probably needed more if you have been lying down throughout your labour. Assisted births may involve the use of forceps, or a ventouse. Forceps are rarely used these days: a tool similar to a pair of tongs is fixed around your baby's head to gently ease him or her out of the birth canal. The ventouse is another tool used to ease the baby from your body. It is a suction device that is attached to the baby's head for gently pulling.

EPISIOTOMY

This is another procedure that is not done so often these days, and involves making an incision between the vagina and perineum to allow more space for the baby to come out.

CAESARIAN SECTION

A Caesarian or C-Section is when you are given either an epidural, or a full anaesthetic, your belly is cut open, and the baby removed. An elective caesarian is one that is planned, for various medical reasons, and often because a previous birth has been a caesarian. However, it is possible to have a vaginal birth after caesarian (VBAC) although you may have to fight hard for it.

An emergency caesarian is one performed, often at the end of a very long labour, or when some other medical issue has been discovered that contraindicates the labour continuing.

If you discover you do need to have a planned caesarian, consider making it as 'natural' as possible. For example, do you want to have your own music playing in the room? Can you ask for your baby to be passed to you directly after the birth, for skin to skin contact, and breastfeeding. Can the room have as few professionals as possible in attendance? Can the lights be dimmed for the birth?

Chapter Nine

ONWARD INTO MOTHERHOOD

"Birth is not only about making babies. Birth is about making mothers - strong, competent, capable mothers who trust themselves and know their inner strength."

Barbara Katz Rothman

"Becoming a mother requires a supreme focus, a profound discipline, and even a kind of warrior spirit."

Naomi Wolfe

MOTHERHOOD IS THE FOUNDATION of human life. The journey of motherhood you are about to embark upon is one of the most rewarding, challenging, and inspiring journeys. However, nothing can prepare you for it. When you are pregnant the entire focus is on the birth; I'm not sure we are even capable at that stage of thinking beyond the birth to conceiving of ourselves as actual mothers. The first 40 days are a time of enormous changes: in yourself, physically and psychologically, in your baby as they grow, in your relationship with the baby's father, and your relationships with the baby's grandparents.

THE POST-NATAL PERIOD

Immediately after the birth is a precious, peaceful time of counting fingers and toes, getting to know your baby, and if you've had it at home, tea and toast in bed. Now you can begin to bond with your baby, and find yourself in your new role as a mother. Be kind to yourself: your body has just gone through an intense physical experience and you may be sore. You will also have some postpartum bleeding, or lochia, which can last for up to six weeks, so prepare yourself by having plenty of heavy duty pads. Your baby may want to feed immediately, or may take some time to latch on. She will probably be quite sleepy for a few hours after the birth.

THE FIRST FEW WEEKS

Let me not beat about the bush, the first few weeks are tough, although they can be wonderful. All your time will be taken up by your precious new arrival, you probably won't be getting much sleep, you may be isolated, and you'll probably feel you haven't got a clue what you're doing. Add to that the well-intentioned advice from family, friends, and people in the street, and your sense of self is more than likely to take a battering. But… everything passes, and the tough bits will be permeated with moments of such heavenly joy, it will be worth it. So, armed with this information, I can only advise you of what a friend wrote in one of our first new baby cards: 'remember, the first six weeks is just survival'. Don't try to take anything on. You don't have anything to prove. Just survive. Sleep when you can, eat when you can, and look after yourselves the best you can.

In traditional cultures in India, the mother was looked after for 40 days after the birth by family, having her meals brought to her and her housework done. Although this is not possible for almost all of us, it is worth bearing in mind. You hear many stories about women who are so proud to have been out in a restaurant the day after giving birth, or having cooked the whole family a three course meal in the first week. I would urge caution, and a strong sense of self-love here.

FROM 'THE WOMAN'S COMFORT BOOK' BY JENNIFER LOUDEN

'Self-care is essential to survival, it is essential as the basis for healthy authentic relationships, it is essential if we honestly want to nurture the people we care about. Self-care is not selfish or self-indulgent. We cannot nurture others from a dry well. We need to take care of our own needs first, then we can give from our surplus, our abundance. When we nurture others from a place of fullness, we feel renewed instead of taken advantage of. And they feel renewed too, instead of guilty. We have something precious to give others when we have been comforting and care for ourselves and building up self-love.'

This is the time to refer to your 'yummy list' and to make some time for you in the fray of caring for a newborn baby. Even if you just create a few minutes each day to listen to a meditation or walk round the garden on your own, it all helps.

BREASTFEEDING

Breastfeeding is the most wonderful way to connect with your baby and to give him or her the best nourishment and nutrition to set him up for life. Breastfeeding isn't as easy or natural as you might think. It can take perseverance and determination, and you may need someone to show you what to do, and help you a bit. The main thing is about getting the baby in the right position for the feed and to make sure they are attached to the nipple correctly. There are breastfeeding counsellors who can help you if you're struggling, and your midwife or health visitor may be able to help. It can take 6-8 weeks to develop a satisfactory breastfeeding relationship with your baby. During this time, it can be very sore on your nipples and extremely time consuming. In addition, your breasts may leak, so you will need breast pads (disposable or washable) and a comfortable breastfeeding bra with drop-down clips. Once breastfeeding is established, it is a breeze. On tap milk, at the right temperature, wherever you are. Just lift your top!

ONGOING BABY CARE

In my experience, many, if not all, mothers have a good instinct at knowing what their babies need. There are many different theories of parenting you can choose from, which change according to the seasons. I always found that I would be going along quite happily until I picked up a baby care book, only to discover my baby wasn't sleeping at the allocated times, or hadn't reached the designated milestones, at which point, I would feel inadequate and like I wasn't doing a very good job at all. If you're feeling unsure and uncertain about what your baby needs, hold her or him, be still together for a few minutes and see if you can work it out between you. With my babies, if they started crying when someone else was holding them, I would always have to take them back and hold them for a while to get a sense of what it was and how I could comfort them. With new babies, it's almost always one of three things: hunger, nappy, need a cuddle. And some babies just seem to cry, regardless. Respond with loving kindness and you'll be fine. Naomi Staedlen in 'What Mother's Do' says, " although it can feel alarming, the 'all-at-sea' feeling is appropriate. Uncertainty is a good starting point for a mother. Through uncertainty, she can begin to learn."

GETTING OUT

Once you're feeling ready, it's good to get out and about and meet other new mothers. Connecting with other mothers will give you the opportunity to swap notes, and feel that you're not alone. It can be quite isolating otherwise, and even though it can be daunting to turn up at your first mother and baby group, I think you will find it more than worth it to share your mothering journey with others.

LOOKING AFTER YOURSELF

- ▶ Take some time each day to listen to a meditation, either on your own or with your baby. Something like a yoga nidra (yoga sleep) can be deeply relaxing, and help you to heal yourself after the birth. You can find guided meditations online or via apps such as the Insight Timer.

- Allow your partner, or any visitors, to look after the baby so you can have a rest or a bath.
- Remember to eat properly. It's so easy to forget, or pass on having lunch when your time is so consumed.
- Whatever your experience of being a mother is, however you are feeling, be kind to yourself.

PART TWO

A BEAUTIFUL COLLECTION OF POSITIVE BIRTH STORIES SPECIALLY CHOSEN TO UPLIFT, INSPIRE YOU AND MAKE YOU LAUGH

There seems to be a conspiracy amongst women to keep the experience of birth to themselves, particularly the good experiences. These stories don't hide anything, are not ashamed of anything, and give you the whole truth, warts and all. Enjoy them, take inspiration from them, and understand the experience of birth.

NUMBER TWO IN MORE WAYS THAN ONE

I may have been on a hospital bed throughout, had several IV drips in my arms, had my legs in stirrups and even a suction cup – but as far as I was concerned, this was more au naturel than I could have dreamed of! "I'd say there's about a 95% chance you will end up with a repeat Caesarean; Trust me, I've had a lot of experience with women like you." Thus said my Obstetrician, with a touch of condescension, about halfway through my pregnancy.

By way of background: I'm a type 1 diabetic – which in a nutshell means I take several insulin injections every day, and in pregnancy have an increased risk of a large baby and early deterioration of the placenta. With my first baby, I was induced at 39 weeks, and despite 48 hours of labour, and 9 cms of dilation, she was delivered by emergency Caesarean, weighing a fairly average 7lb 14oz.

Much to the confusion of some of my friends, I have always been keen on having a baby the 'natural' way. By which I don't mean at home, in the ocean, in silence, or in a crop circle with chanting elders, but just vaginally. I figure, it's the one unifying experience that we share with the earliest female homo sapiens, and that to me, is kind of cool. But of course the method of birth is all really a footnote in the general motherhood experience. However long the labour, however scarce the pain relief – it is nothing compared to the challenge of being a mother.

So that was what I told myself when the doctor gave his definitive pronouncement. He grew all the more convinced as I entered the third trimester and had growth scans that showed the baby getting big. Quite big. VERY BIG! By 34 weeks, some of his measurements were the average size for a gestation of 42 weeks. Being a rather smallish lady of 5 ft, I looked like a small person attached to the side of a massive beach ball. So I said mea culpa (too much chocolate, not enough insulin…), and resigned myself to a scheduled C-section in week 38. As it happened my toddler was turning two in week 35, so we planned a big bash for her and I put off any baby prep until afterwards. The party came and went, and I began to think about fetching the newborn kit down from the attic. I'd got through washing the first batch of newborn bodysuits, when on the Friday I came down with a bit of the old tummy-bug. How unpleasant is that when you're heavily pregnant?? After a day of unpleasantries, I was going to bed feeling better but – god damn Braxton Hicks, why do they have to start now? And then, at 1am, something went twang. "What was that??" I heard myself saying aloud. A few moments later, when nothing more happened, I dismissed it as one of those pregnancy things, the baby probably kicked my kidneys or something. I rolled over, and … gush! Thirty seconds later my husband was a flurry of towels and telephones. "For god sakes, honey, STAY ON THE LOO! I don't need you leaking all over the carpet! I'll pack your hospital bag." Well, he did, and you can imagine what obscure stuff I ended up with…

We called the hospital, and they told us to come in at once. Having spent two days in labour with my first, and given that contractions had not even started, I couldn't imagine we didn't have time to wait for my mother-in-law to drive down from Norwich to watch the toddler. But the hospital said 'come now', so we had to call on a neighbour to come round And just as well. By the time we got to hospital, contractions were well and truly established, and only three minutes apart. By the time I was in the bed and they'd found my notes, read them, found the insulin drip, found the glucose drip, found the fetal heart monitor, and of course found the 14 veins they needed to stick all the drips into – well by then I was very, very, very keen on the idea of an epidural! "Yes of course, as soon as the Anaesthetist is out of surgery, we'll send him right in," they told me.

In no time – and no epidural – I realised I'd gotten into the pushing stage. To be blunt, I knew this because I poo'd. And while I would have cringed to think about it beforehand, once it happened, I though "oh well, let's embrace that method of getting on with it". I'm glad I did, because it proved immensely effective. I had about two or three contractions of pushing, with my legs up in stirrups – and out the baby slipped.

At 4.30am, three and a half hours after my waters broke, baby Ben was born. For all that he was a month early, he was still 8lbs 14oz - a strapping lad. He was whisked off to Special Care, where he remained for a few days - mainly to stabilise his blood sugars, but also to tackle a bout of jaundice that developed subsequently. I was in a complete daze, still hardly believing it had all happened, as fast and as thrillingly as it did (ok, not an adjective you'd expect – I can't explain it, but it really was thrilling). The baby down the corridor who'd resulted from it all was almost an afterthought.

I was pleased to discover I could get up and take a shower immediately. When I emerged from the shower room, I spotted Dr Zanussi (aka Dr You-are-SO-gonna-end-up-with-a-slice-and-dice) at the other end of the hallway. "DR ZANUSSI!!!", I hollered, "GUESS WHAT I JUST DID??". To his credit, he was very congratulatory, and only joked a little bit about how the baby had cheated him of his caesarean appointment.

So I feel I've learned a few things: Subsequent births can be speedy; Birth with no pain relief works for me (I don't believe it works for everyone, and nobody should get a medal for it, but I was glad in hindsight that the anaesthetist was tied up); The doctors can always be proven wrong; And to be blunt, because this is important, nothing brings on labour as effectively as the runs. Sorry, but that's the unpalatable truth!

Dina

THE RHESUS NEGATIVE BIRTH

After 2 nice easy pregnancy/births - one in hospital and one at home you would expect a third to be as trouble free!!! Ha ha ha!. First attempt at number 3 ended at 9 weeks (blighted ovum), 2nd visit at 7 weeks and 3rd was a no heartbeat at 9 weeks job. I basically gave up, despite having been told by the Gyny that there wasn't anything wrong with me! Obviously the man upstairs had other ideas and I finally became pregnant again 4 months after the last attempt.

I was watched carefully for the first 12 weeks by the Early Pregnancy unit - and was then turned over to the arms of my lovely community midwife, who then promptly told me that she would be away for the last 2 months of my pregnancy. Her replacement turned out to be a real little Miss Worry-pants! Every twinge and slightly more than normal discharge was deemed to be something dire - and she also decided that my bump wasn't growing when I was 35 weeks..so I spent a boring morning stuck on a monitor in the hospital finally being told nothing was wrong with the baby (I could have told them that!). I suffered really badly from DSP (pelvic pain) - only eased by a wonderful physio and remembering to do my exercises! I spent the whole of Christmas/New Year having pretty ghastly Braxton Hicks - not helped by the baby swivelling round all the time. I really was totally fed up by the time due day came around- the boys had gone back to school and I spent all day whinging and moaning until DH (darling husband) suggested I do the school run to get me out of the house! It was yucky and rainy and the drive takes about 20 mins. On the way back - feeling more road ragey than normal I suddenly had a contraction when I was negotiating a mini roundabout! Ouch!

4.20pm Got home - Mum was there for some reason - said I thought I felt something might be happening, but by the time we'd had a cup of tea and a chat things died down.

5.30pm Feeling a need to be alone I went upstairs with the laptop and started reading my email - I had just read one from my friend Caro saying to please let her know when I started labour...when I had another contraction. I grabbed the birth ball from the bathroom and sat rocking on it whilst reading – wondering whether to post something or not.. decided that my need for the toilet was more urgent!

6.00ish Locked myself in the toilet whilst body did the 'emptying itself in preparation' job whilst I fended off my 5 year old who wanted to come in to see me!! I asked him to get Daddy - but he thought he would wander off into his bedroom to play on his Gameboy instead. Finally got the 7 year old to hear me and DH came after what felt like hours (I'm sure it was only a few minutes really - but I was panicking!).

6.30pm DH told to ring hospital and get Mum to come back and pick the boys up. I am now rocking on the birth ball in the bathroom in between loo trips and having to concentrate on breathing - suddenly remember what labour is like and wishing I could just postpone and think about it tomorrow.

Midwife is contacted and rings back - she is in the next town and it is rush hour - would be over as soon as she could but it may be 3/4 hour - I think I said something like 'I neeedd gas and airrrrr' and not much else (I always read other peoples drug–free births with awe.'

6.45pm DH helps to put the TENs machine on - I put it on pretty high and enjoy the strange throbbing. It works for a while as a good distraction technique if nothing else!

Midwife arrives in 15 minutes (no idea how she managed that!), flips through my notes and birth plan and apologises but says please can she just do one examination with me on my back on the floor, which is horrible. I am 4 cms - thought I was doing better than.

7.30ish My technique switches from the birth ball to sitting on the loo rocking through contractions - and as they peaked I stood up, rocking more intensely and visualising myself as a small boat riding over a very large wave. After about half and hour of this the sea was feeling decidedly choppy..and I needed to shout mayday! Bring in that gas and air.

8pm So there I am on the toilet, TENs in one hand, gas and air in the other, wires and tubes everywhere - thinking 'Hey it's so natural this homebirth lark!' Midwife is eating her tea outside the bathroom (DH was making himself useful!) and keeping out of my way as requested. We would have a quick chat between contractions - but she knew when not to speak fortunately! Despite not having met her before we seemed to jell pretty well, and certainly acted on all the things I had asked in my plan - even giving me my homeopathy (highly recommend Arnica during and after labour).

8.30pm After a while I felt like I was getting to the point of double peaked contractions without much of a break - and my bottom was getting numb from sitting on the loo all that time (how do men stay in the loo for hours????) so Theresa suggested a change of scene - which was a real palaver as you imagine the sight of me clanking across the landing with the canister, wires, sick bucket etc etc!

I plant myself, standing at the end of the bed - where I can grip the gas and air mouthpiece in my mouth and grip onto the end of the bedrail and rock back and forth during contractions - they are really getting almost too much more and I feel myself focusing more and more into myself and blocking out the outside world. For some reason DH comes upstairs and says 'Hey Raiders of the Lost Ark has just started - shall I put it on the telly in here?' I managed to say 'Noooo' as I have the comical thought of giving birth in front of Harrison Ford.

Contractions tumbling one into the other - I am quietly sobbing and then want to be sick - grab the bucket but instead of heaving I just breathe loudly through the next contraction which feels like it is a triple peaking one and suddenly my waters break. There is a lot of action behind me as Theresa catches most of it in a dish she has brought with her - telling me it is clear and not blood or meconium stained (phew!). The baby suddenly seems to drop down and is pressing down on my cervix and the contractions start to change. I am leaning over the edge of the bed with my bottom in the air and Theresa is frantically phoning the second midwife to come now. I have a slight lull where the contractions are pushy but still painful - I am not pushing in any way as I feel this is transition and not quite full second stage. I am moaning quietly into a pillow by this point and thinking 'Oh nooo - I can't stop this now and go to bed - it really will have to come out.'

Then all of a sudden my body simply wants to get this baby outta there! I don't have to push - it is just one huge downward urge - I bury my head and moan something like 'nnuggggghhhh!' as the baby bundles his way out - Theresa is having to move a large pile of dirty laundry out of the way behind me and chuck more inco pads down as the head appears. She quickly feels around the neck to find his hand is up by his chin and as DH and the second midwife appear in the doorway he slithers out. I am so into myself with intenseness of it all that I don't realised he has come out completely - DH has to tell me!!!

A loud lusty yell from the baby lets me know he is okay - I stand up and have the baby passed up between my legs and placed on a towel in front of me (I am feeling too wobbly myself as planned) and I look down at the scene underneath me - sort of resembled the Battle of the Somme I remember thinking!!! My blood loss was noted as 200mls.

I had opted for a natural third stage, and within 4 minutes I feel another painless contraction and the placenta drops out - it is huge and complete - so no worries there. The baby in the meantime is perfect - although he was born with blue feet and hands that gradually start to pink up after about 15 minutes - so his apgar is 9 to start with and 10. I am quickly washed down and wrapped in a towel and sat on the bed - and baby is snuggled up with me - he is perfect, gorgeous, 8lbs 11oz with sweet dimples in both cheeks! The midwives clear all the mess away - 2 towels grabbed from the bathroom in a hurry are deemed too hideous to bother washing - and the rest had been caught on the inco pads. I decline a bath - and finally get a cup of tea - DH having made everyone else one and had forgotten to make me one! I was starving and there wasn't any food leftover from teatime ('Well you weren't hungry then were you?') so I get him to raid the cake tin instead - the best piece of Chocolate cake I've ever tasted!!

The midwives quickly took a blood test from me (I am rhesis negative) and filled in their notes in another room (so I could concentrate on the baby - as written in my notes) and I reflected on how everyday and really rather matter of fact it had all been! The baby latched on like a pro - and we all settled down for the night (after the obligatory phone calls) with our special little gift lying between us!

Caroline

THE PRIVATE HOSPITAL BIRTH

After having two quite two very straight forward and normal births but also very medical and intervening, I felt I hadn't achieved the 'perfect birth' (if there is such a thing yet) and was very keen to make what was probably going to be my last baby a good birth. With my first daughter I was very young and felt I had to obey all hospital staff and had that horrible experience of having to lie down flat with bright hospital lights and very little support with lots of people dictating to me, the whole experience was daunting and traumatic and even then I felt that there must be another way.....

Six years later when having Olivia with my husband, he knew my concerns and how I felt about my first experience so we decided early on that maybe it was the NHS that was the problem and booked into the Portland. However halfway through I felt uneasy about it and felt I hadn't chosen the right hospital, it was still very medical and I didn't agree with a lot of their values, picking the day your baby is born etc etc, I didn't feel this was going to give me the right birth experience for me so I opted out after finding out about the Hemel birthing centre. I booked in there but I had a slow starting labour and after spending the whole day there instead of sending me home they send me to Luton and Dunstable hospital (and I stupidly went!) where they induced me which seems ridiculous now as I wasn't in that much pain and it was 2 weeks before my due date, they could have sent me home to wait for things to start properly.

With Sienna I felt I finally got my perfect birth experience, I booked into John and Lizzies, a private hospital in London with a very different attitude to the Portland, they promote natural birth, listen to the mother, don't intervene unless asked, enjoy having the whole family in to stay afterwards etc etc (in hindsight I should have just had her at home but just totally lacked the confidence!). I had a water birth there with candlelight and lots of fantastic support. The midwives were always there but somehow managed to make it feel like it was just Marvin and I in the room. It felt like being at home and I can't rate the place or the midwives there enough. Unfortunately Sienna had breathing difficulties afterwards and we had to be transferred to The Portland which was not such a nice experience (they were unsupportive and rude there!) as John and Lizzies does not have a special care unit, So we nearly had the perfect whole experience!!!

Lauren

THE 'BIRTHING FROM WITHIN' BIRTH

When I was pregnant with my first child, aged 25, I felt afraid, alone, daunted and unprepared for this rite of passage which lay before me. This was despite reading everything I could get my hands on. I knew the facts, but I did not know if, how, I could give birth. The doctor and midwife team knew the exact proportions of my blood and urine, and listened to the butterfly beat of my unborn's heart, but knew nothing of my heart, my deepest fears, those things which would have probably more impact on the birthing process than anything that they were testing. There was not time. It was not their job. I knew I needed to prepare, but how? Asking questions of those who had gone before me was a start. But their unconsciousness of their own birthing processes created as many new worries for me as it gave reassurance. And so I continued to read, haunting myself with visions of Caesarians and episiotomy. My husband would come in from work to find a sobbing wreck curled up in bed, and pleaded with me not to read any more. But I needed to know: what is birth, how can I do it?

Fast-forward a year. My birth was a textbook delivery at home: a powerful, erotic, spiritual, grounding, exhilarating, profound experience. But this was not inevitable. I truly believe that I gained the physical (through yoga) and spiritual and emotional (through Birthing From Within) preparation that allowed me to step out of the way and allow the birth to happen.

My favourite moment from that first birth, my only son, was the lion's roar which came from me. The power of my voice, coming with full force from my belly, a roaring-screaming-spine tingling- gut wrenching primal noise – this is my power. This is my woman-power, hear me roar. A moment later I worried that my teenage sister, asleep next door would have heard and be terrified of the act of birth. But for that moment, that pure moment, I was there , on all fours, truly grounded in my own power. I do not know how it would have been had I not prepared. I know other friends who have prepared and yet had hard, traumatic births. But I believe strongly, that the more preparation one does, the less one leaves up to chance, the less one has left to come up in the maelstrom of the birth process. Birth is a messy business; it is deeply tied up with our feelings about ourselves, our families, our partners, our sexual natures, our feminine bodies, ourselves as creative or spiritual beings, our mortality - there is a lot to be looked at. Making space for deep reflection on these issues during pregnancy, when we are naturally slowing down and becoming more emotionally sensitive, can only be beneficial.

Lucy

THE DOCTOR'S BIRTH

From the beginning of my pregnancy with our first son Ben I planned to have a natural birth with as little intervention as possible. I was even considering a home birth as my pregnancy progressed well without any complications. First doubts came when I started my new job as a doctor in neonatology in a hospital in East London. This was a very deprived area with a large amount of complicated deliveries which I had to attend. I was shocked by the amount of medical intervention, lack of choices for the women and very poor communication skills from the midwives. At this point I was quite scared of delivering my own child in the UK and thought about going home to Germany to have Ben there. Nevertheless, my pregnancy continued to be uncomplicated and I managed to work in my stressful job until 34 weeks of pregnancy.

When I reached 38 weeks I saw yet another different community midwife who was not sure if Ben was in a breech position and thought that I looked small. We went to the QE2 hospital in Welwyn Garden City for a scan which showed that Ben was well but a bit on the small side. From then on I was monitored more closely in the community with weekly appointments which made me more nervous rather than reassuring me. I knew from work that the more monitoring there was the more likely there would be complications. My due date approached and I was still very fit, doing regular yoga and riding my bike to the midwife appointment. Now I was told that Ben's head was not engaged and that I should walk a lot which I did. No signs of labour for the next week. There was another midwife appointment at 9 days past my due date and induction became a more and more likely scenario of which I was very afraid, knowing all the possible complications. During this appointment the midwife was again unsure if Ben was now in a breech position and thought that his head was still not engaged. We were sent to the hospital again for another scan and to book an induction.

At 10 days after my due date we went to the hospital and a scan confirmed that Ben's head was in the correct position and engaged but that he had not grown much in the last 3 weeks. One of the hospital midwives did a CTG (Cardiotarcography, a technical means of recording the fetal heartbeat and the uterine contractions during pregnancy) which showed that Ben was otherwise well. Afterwards one of the registrars then came to see us and wanted to induce labour on the same day as I was already 10 days overdue. I was not keen on that at all, especially since the doctor did not really explain any risks and benefits nor give us a different option. After confirming with her and the midwife that there was no danger for Ben to wait longer I said that I preferred to try a membrane sweep and go home and did not want to be induced. The registrar was not very convinced but the midwife was very supportive and performed the membrane sweep. I was told to come back the next day for an induction We went home that day and watched movies, as well as going to a restaurant and I tried to take my mind of the induction. I woke up at around 3 am and felt some slight abdominal discomfort which continued to come and go. Happy that contractions had now finally started and I did not need an induction I tried to go back to sleep as I thought that labour might take some time. I told my partner in the early morning and now we were both up and not able to sleep anymore. Contractions became stronger and more regular. I spent time cooking some light food, sat on my yoga mat and the birthing ball and started my yoga breathing with contractions. As advised by the hospital I took a bath and some paracetamol. By 3 pm my contractions were regular and lasted for about 1 minute. Chris talked to the hospital who said we could come for an assessment.

In the hospital I was told that I was only 2 cm dilated and the midwife wanted to put me on a CTG monitor, as well as getting one of the doctors to start the induction now. Again I asked if that was really necessary and said that I would prefer to go home. I did not see the point to induce labour which had already started or wait in hospital for possibly 2 or 3. Back at home I took another bath and was by now getting quite tired as contractions had almost been going for a whole day. Having heard that it might take another couple of days was very discouraging. At 9 pm we then went back to the hospital as I was exhausted.

Luckily, the midwives had changed and we got an excellent midwife who was going to stay with us for the next 8 hours. Another assessment and now I was 4-5 cm dilated and was in established labour, so finally no more talk of induction. The midwife asked about our birth preferences and agreed that I should continue to have an as natural birth as possible. She advised us to just ignore all the induction and scan excitement from the last couple of days and rather focus on the uncomplicated pregnancy I had and that I was generally fit and well. She did write a short CTG which confirmed that Ben was well and coping with the contractions. We were lucky and had a room with a birthing pool which was filled for me. As soon as I entered the pool I felt much more relaxed and the contractions seemed less painful. After some time the midwife suggested to try gas and air which worked very well and which I then kept using almost until Ben's delivery. From now on labour progressed faster and by 1 am I was already 8 cm dilated. Our midwife stayed with us and I remember her as a supportive and unobtrusive presence at the side of the birthing pool in which I was floating. She regularly checked Ben's heart beat, my temperature and made sure that the water remained warm. Unlike other hospitals the QE2 in Welwyn Garden City has no policy which restricts the amount of time spent in the pool which was very good for me as I stayed in the water for about 8 hours in total. We were asked if I wanted to deliver Ben in the water. We had not actually planned to do so but as I was so comfortable in the pool we decided to do so. In the early morning I was told by our midwife to listen to my body and start pushing when I felt I was ready to push.

Being relaxed in the water I was able to do that and pushed when I felt ready to do so. Having only seen medicalised birth in hospital I was surprised that there was no intervention or perineal support given to me. At 5.50 am I was able to deliver Ben's head and then his body without any aid in the water where he was received by the midwife and then put onto my chest. As he did not cry immediately another midwife took him to a resuscitaire where he got some initial help with breathing which he did very soon. My midwife helped me out of the pool onto a bed where the placenta was delivered after an injection into my leg. Ben was put back onto my chest as soon as he started breathing and I was able to hold and feed him.

After a shower Ben and I were transferred to the post-natal ward where we stayed until the evening and then went back home the same day. During this time friendly midwives and health care assistants helped us with feeding and explained what to expect after. Looking back at this in the end very nice and natural birth experience I have come to realise how important it is to have a good and supportive midwife. Having some medical knowledge I was also in a position to say no to the proposed induction and wait for Ben to be born when he was ready to come. I think that every woman should be given choices and sufficient explanations to make those decisions rather than being put into a "delivery machinery" which makes complications more likely.

Franziska

THE 'IT STARTED IN THE SUPERMARKET BIRTH'

The pregnancy was not too bad – I was quite sick to start with but kept up with swimming and cycling the whole way through and apart from feeling terribly tired until the last trimester, really enjoyed it. The last bit was wonderful, especially after I stopped work. I felt really well and enjoyed pottering at home. I tried not to wish away the time til the birth and Keith and I had a lovely time - meals together with this fabulous sense of anticipation. The weather was lovely in the weeks before too so I was lunching in the garden in the sun – it was great! We had decided on a home birth as I was keen to have the minimum of intervention in the birth as this is best for the baby (assuming all goes normally).

We also thought it would be a much nicer experience if we could have the baby at home rather than in hospital. However, we remained open minded that there was a good chance, with a first baby, that we might end up in hospital anyway (often first labours are inefficient and need some helping along). Given the pitiful service the NHS offered we decided to pay for private midwives and went to Birthrites and we were allocated two midwives to look after us – Melody Weig was my main one and Annie Francis was the back up -they shared the antenatal and postnatal visits.

On the Monday of the week Georgia arrived, I started to get a bit tetchy as I had done most of the things I had wanted to get done before she arrived – it was hard not to start to be impatient. That night I had some contractions but they died out in the morning when I got up so Keith went off to work and nothing happened during the day (that was very frustrating). The same happened on Tuesday night although I had a bit of a show which suggested things really were happening. However, again, in the morning things died down but I did continue to have contractions on and off during the day. Our midwives had told us to keep ignoring the contractions until we couldn't anymore because they could come and go on and off for weeks before true labour really started. I went shopping and was having contractions on and off round Sainsburys!

The contractions continued but erratically for the evening and we went to bed. I tried to sleep but couldn't so we got up and tried out the tens machine as a practice for when the labour really started (!). I was sick a few times and this continued on and off over the evening/night. By 2am we realised that this was the real thing (my contractions were 5 mins apart). We rang Melody who suggested we got in the birthing pool. I was not amused at this as I thought she was just playing for time to avoid having to come out (the rational effects of labour!!). – I was worried I was not advanced enough to get in the pool and that it would therefore slow the contractions again. Keith and I agreed we would try the pool but if things slowed down I would get out again.

The pool (which was in the middle of the dining room) was ready by 3.30ish so I got in and things speeded up immediately – my contractions were 3 minutes apart. I remember this lovely phase where classical music was playing and the candles were burning and between contractions I was looking out of the window at the lilac tree in blossom in the garden and the dawn breaking and Keith was quietly lying on the sofa timing the contractions. At 5am we agreed we would ring Melody at 6am (believing I would be labouring for all of Thursday as well). At 5.10 am I told Keith to get Melody. My waters broke at about 5.40 – it was an amazing sensation – I felt and heard the pop (like a balloon full of water). Keith checked the pool and there was no sign that the amniotic fluid was anything but clear. Things really got serious then. The contractions were almost constant and very strong. I was retching a lot too. Melody arrived at 5.45 and eventually I agreed for her to check how dilated I was (I was worried that I would only be 3 cms or something) I was 8cms ish and she said I was in transition. I didn't really believe her as I had imagined it would take much longer to get to that stage. This stage and the pushing stage was the hardest thing I think I have ever had to do. It was painful in a way that is impossible to describe – my pelvis felt like it was going to burst and I knew there was only one way to escape the pain and that was to go through it and surrender to it. I couldn't really even have gas and air by that point as it can make you feel sick and I was already being sick. Keith found this stage very hard too and went into the kitchen for a bit and made a cup of tea.

Melody was excellent in helping me to give in to the pain and push productively and at 6.59am on 25 April 2002 Georgia shot into the world. She did not crown - she just came out head, shoulders – the whole lot in one contraction. The one thing I will never forget is that as she came out I could feel the difference between her face and the back of her head – I felt her profile go by on the way out – it was amazing and something I wouldn't have felt if I had had an epidural. Her rapid arrival took Melody by surprise and Georgia sunk to the bottom of the pool and Melody had to pick her up from the bottom!

Melody had got Keith to whack up the central heating - Georgia and I said hello in the pool then they dried Georgia and warmed her up – she had done her bit by getting into the right position just before the birth (she had had her back to my back up to a short while before the birth) which I think made the labour so efficient. I also think the nights of contractions before also helped do some of the work so the labour lasted 13 hours or so. We had a cuddle on the sofa and Georgia was weighed (7lb exactly). Then we had a bath together and Melody washed my hair for me and then we went to bed. Keith made us bacon sandwiches and Georgia had a bit at the breast. We cracked open the champers but I only managed a few sips (not like me I know!)

What an overwhelming experience – our daughter is just beautiful but nothing prepares you for parenthood – your hormones are all over the place and you are just flailing around in the dark as you don't know whether her cry means she is hungry, dirty, tired… or she is just crying! There are no rules and no-one knows your child better than you (and you don't know her!). There is no objectively right answer to any given issue so you just muddle along using trial and error! Of course there is also a totally all-consuming desire to do the right thing for this miraculous creature. It is pretty hard to achieve when you are not sure what the right thing is!!

Everyone agrees though that she is just beautiful!

Joanna

AND FINALLY.. MY OWN BIRTH STORIES

When I became pregnant with my first child, I knew that I wanted to give birth naturally, preferably at home, and preferably into water. I always had a strong opinion about letting gravity take effect, and birthing in an upright position. My husband was absolutely horrified, but after a couple of meetings with our fantastic midwife he felt happy to go along with the plan. When we asked her after several visits, "What do you actually do at the birth?" her reply was, "Oh, I'll just sit in the corner and drink coffee." Obviously there was a little more to it than that, but she managed to convey her absolute conviction of the body's ability to birth without intervention. Little did Simon know quite how minimal that intervention would be. Not only did he cut the cord on all four of our children, he was also my sole supporter for two of their births. These are my stories, and my inspiration for this book. By the time I was 39 weeks pregnant, I was absolutely desperate to have my first baby. I could be pregnant no more! And I really wanted to meet her (we knew it was a girl). So, my husband and I had planned a full weekend of bringing on baby activity.

Thursday was to be pineapple day – but pineapples appeared to be scarce at this time of year. On Friday evening we were going for a curry and for Saturday we had planned hot sex. Sadly for my husband, the baby had other ideas for him, and we never made it to the Saturday. On Friday afternoon I had visited a friend with an 8 week old baby and the babies had a bit of a cuddle (mine on the inside, hers on the outside), and I think this may have triggered something. We went for the curry as planned, ordered our food, Simon had a nice cool beer waiting for him, then suddenly, 'whoosh'. I felt something watery gush between my legs. Luckily it was a small, containable amount! I told Simon that I thought my waters had broken and he blanched even whiter than he did when I told him I was pregnant. I rushed to the ladies in the restaurant and there was further gushing. I was pretty sure this was it. I went back to the table and, not wanting to miss out on a good curry arranged to have a takeaway.

We took it home, called Katrina, who said to have a glass of wine, enjoy the curry, and wait and see what happens. Not much did happen. We went to bed. I had period type pains throughout the night. By about

8am, I felt I couldn't stay in bed any longer. We called the midwife again and she came out. As soon as she arrived, everything stopped completely, so she left, and let us get on with it. (It's interesting to note that this was the second midwife who we did not know so well). The day continued, with occasional discomfort in my abdomen, but nothing to speak of. By about lunchtime, having spent all morning wandering around the house, listening to music, and generally relaxing, we decided to put on a Woody Allen film. Whilst watching this, the chuckling must have had an effect as it was around this time that I was fairly sure proper labour was coming on (after all, you don't really know with your first baby – or, truth be told, second and subsequent). I started to feel sensations across my belly, and tried the tens machine.

There is a photo of me around this time on a beautiful sunny day sitting in our little patio garden hooked up to the tens machine (which seemed like more of a distraction than anything) reading a book. I can't remember what book it was, and I'm not sure I was taking any of it in. We then called the midwife again and they both arrived shortly after I had climbed into the pool. I spent the next several hours wallowing in warm water. I don't think I really believed that I was having an actual baby and it took a leap of imagination and faith to believe that this being was coming through me. Once I had reached that point, aided by cooing over a tiny babygro, everything progressed much quicker. However, subtle as ever, my midwife, Katrina, suggested I may need to go to the loo. Now, having given birth in water three times, I know that 'going to the loo' is no more than a matter of releasing into the water, but it was her subtle way of suggesting that my body may feel more comfortable with the 'opening' sensation when on the loo. She was right. No sooner had I sat down, and the midwives popped downstairs, than the head began to crown. We called them back. I slowly shuffled back to the birthing room, where I knelt on all fours, and within a few moments, the head was out. By this time, I was really concentrating on pushing the body out, but Simon was really excited to see the head, and I told him to 'calm down'. I still had more to do! But not very much. Another few moments and out came the body. Katrina passed my beautiful Naomi through my legs so I could hold her. Nothing could describe the wonder, ecstasy and elation at holding my little one. I knelt back and put her to my breast whilst we waited for the cord to stop pulsing. Simon cut the cord. I gave the baby to her Daddy, had a shower, and within half an hour we were snuggled up in our own bed with tea, toast and our new and precious baby.

My next and subsequent stories won't take so long…Each birth halved in time between onset of labour and delivery. My first took 6 hours. With my second baby, Hannah, I was in bed, at night, 39 weeks pregnant. It was 2.30am and my waters gently broke. I told Simon, then went downstairs to do some yoga, relaxed and got into a good frame of mind, then went back to bed until about 4am when I really felt the openings. (That's what I like to call what are usually known as contractions – it's so much more helpful to visualise your body opening with each sensation, rather than contracting). Eventually, I could lie down no longer. I got up, and started padding around the house. By 5am, the midwives, Katrina and Melanie, had arrived and we chatted and laughed whilst they drank coffee, and I leaned against the furniture at increasingly regular intervals to moan and take deep breaths. The lights were dim, the house was quiet and it was all quite lovely. At some point, about an hour or so later, Katrina suggested that if I was going to use the birth pool, I'd better get upstairs now. She and Melanie had just been leaving me to it. There had been no examinations or intrusions, but from observation alone, they knew that I had dilated far enough that the baby was soon to be born.

We all traipsed upstairs (me, two at a time – great for opening the pelvis) and I hopped…well, actually, more like lumbered, into the pool. I had little time for wallowing as things started hotting up pretty quickly. At some point I leant forward onto the side of the pool, felt some very strong abdominal sensations, at which point Katrina said, "You can lean down and pick the baby up." I must confess, I didn't even know I'd had her.

Again, very calmly, "You can lean down and pick the baby up". I looked down, and there was my beautiful Hannah. I scooped her up, out of the water, and held her in my arms, until I was ready to get out of the pool. At some point during all this, I had phoned my parents to come and look after Naomi. As Hannah was born, at around 7am, she cried. Simultaneously, Naomi (now aged 18 months) awoke, and my parents put their key in the lock.

So… Leila was born in around one and a half hours. Again, I was 39 weeks pregnant. Again, in the middle of the night (so much more convenient when you have other children). Again, my waters broke first. But this time, it all progressed much, much quicker. By the time I realised I was in full on labour, and phoned Katrina, I was minutes away from having the 'pushy' sensations which meant the baby was imminent. Simon called her back to hurry her along, and check if it would be ok for me to climb into the pool. She said, "Yes", and Simon (now quite the expert) escorted me into the next bedroom and helped. Within seconds, the "pushy" sensations became stronger. Somewhere in the back of my memory was a recollection of the 'candle breath', taught at a distant NCT class, and intended to prevent things progressing if you're not ready (or something like that). I made a vain attempt to do this, so that I didn't give birth without Katrina being there, but very soon realised that it was futile: this baby was coming. A couple of rushes (this is what 'contractions' are known as by the inspirational American midwife, Ina May Gaskin) later, and I felt down between my legs, only to feel the top of her head emerging. Katrina was still on her way. It was an icy black night in February, and she'd had to deice her car. I said to Simon, "She's coming." His platitude, "Yes…I know…" suggested he thought I meant the midwife. "No, I can feel the baby's head." He blanched, and sheer panic flashed across his pale face, but for moments only, as he gathered himself to be strong for me and the baby. Moments later I squatted back, and a chubby faced Leila gently escaped from my body. At the same time, the phone rang. Katrina was at the door. Simon announced, "She's here!" Katrina thought it odd that he was quite so excited about her arrival, but it was soon revealed that Simon was actually referring to the baby. We cut the cord, cleaned up, had tea and toast in bed, and snoozed a little until Naomi and Hannah (now 3 ½ and 2) came in to meet their new sister in the morning.

Number four was exceptionally quick. It was a boy, and he was a week late, although it felt like two weeks as I had been expecting to have him at 39 weeks, like the girls. I'd already had a false alarm the weekend before when Katrina ended up sleeping on our sofa overnight, but nothing had happened. So, when I woke in the night, around about ten to two, feeling slightly uncomfortable, I got up and went to the loo, thinking nothing of it. I got back into bed, but within moments realised that this was it. I woke Simon up: "I'm pretty sure I'm having the baby". He phoned Katrina. She was on her way immediately. By about 2.15, my waters broke and at the same time I had a huge rush. Simon decided to take me through to the birthing room. I hung around by the edge of the pool, spaced, and a couple of huge rushes later, Joseph (we later discovered, 9lb 4oz) made his appearance. His head came first, and with a gentle push, his body swiftly followed. We had no sterile equipment so couldn't cut the cord. Luckily, I had recently read a couple of articles about Lotus birth in both Juno and The Mother magazines. (This is where the cord is not cut so the placenta remains connected to the baby until it drops off naturally. This can take a couple of weeks and you carry it around in a bowl, with your new baby). Now, this wasn't what I was planning, but at least I was aware that it wouldn't be a problem to leave the cord and placenta until professional assistance arrived. After I got out of the pool, I handed the baby, and placenta in bowl (surprisingly heavy), to Simon whilst I showered. We then got back into bed to wait for Katrina and Natalie. Hannah (now 3½) woke up calling for Mummy. Simon brought her in, she said, "Hello" to her new little brother, and went back to bed until morning! Our midwives arrived one hour after the birth to help with cord cutting and to do all the necessary checks on mother and baby, and left us about an hour later to get some kip. We all dozed off, to be greeted in the morning by one slightly bemused (Leila, now 19 months) and two very excited big sisters. My births have been the most transformative, empowering and ecstatic experiences of my life. I hope my story inspires you, gives you faith in your ability to birth your baby, and sets you out on the journey of motherhood in strength and wonder.

Caroline

APPENDIX

Birth Plan

Where? (Home, hospital, environment in general)

When? (When is your ideal time – when other children asleep? After work?!)

Who? (Who do you want to be present? What do you think you'd like them to do?)

How? (Position, water, massage, music, candles etc etc.)

Communicate your birth plan to your birth partner, midwife, and anyone else you want to involve in your birth.

The Three Pledge Promise of the Pregnant Mother

1. I will honour myself and my body whilst I am pregnant, and beyond.

2. I will focus only on positive birth stories.

3. I will take charge of my birth experience.

Signed ───────────────────────────

RESOURCES

FURTHER READING

Childbirth without Fear by Grantly Dick-Read

New Active Birth by Janet Balaskas

Birth and Breastfeeding by Michel Odent

Your Best Birth by Ricki Lake

Spiritual Midwifery by Ina May Gaskin

Birth Your Way by Sheila Kitzinger

Yoga for Pregnancy and Birth by Uma Dinsmore-Tuli

Blooming Birth by Lucy Atkins

Gas and Air by Jill Dawson and Margo Daly

Gentle Birth Method by Gowri Motha

Bountiful, Beautiful, Blissful by Gurmukh

USEFUL PUBLICATIONS

Juno Magazine

Green Parent

USEFUL WEBSITES

www.aims.org.uk

www.yoursmaternally.co.uk

www.inamay.com

www.activebirthcentre.com

www.nct.org.uk

www.netmums.com

www.hypnobirthing.co.uk

www.mumsnet.com

www.homebirth.org.uk

This book promises to:

- Inform you about natural childbirth and your choices for pregnancy and birth.
- Empower you to take control of your birth experience.
- Inspire you towards a natural and wonderful birth, and entry into motherhood.

About the Author

Caroline Murray studied social science and social work at Coventry University, graduating in the mid '90's. She practiced as a social worker for 10 years, working with children and families in both the state and voluntary sectors, teaching the social work module at Lambeth College, and training social workers on placement. She left social work to try her hand at restaurant managing, book selling and running a holistic health centre, before starting her own domestic cleaning company. Meeting her husband at a business networking event, she quickly became pregnant, and committed to becoming a full-time mother and homemaker, going on to have a further three children. All birthed at home, she is amply qualified to write this book, and determined to impart what she has learnt to others. The journey of motherhood has inspired her to write, and she has had articles published in Juno Magazine and local NCT magazines, relating to motherhood and birth. Caroline is a committed yogini, having practiced yoga in various forms for over twenty years.

CPSIA information can be obtained
at www.ICGtesting.com
Printed in the USA
LVHW081453280120
645066LV00019B/1742